Praise for *Separate Rooms*

'An Italian novel of imperfect love and urgent grief'
New York Times

'A novel of dignified beauty'
Observer

'A masterly piece of writing, rich with insight and detail, and a curiously moving optimism'
Gay Times

'Tondelli's was a meticulous talent, precise and particular, his writing full of nicely observed detail and an almost microscopic view of everyday things and feelings'
Financial Times

'A classic in Italy: a story of love and youth and pain that will have you clutching at your heart. I want everyone to read it; I want to press it into people's hands. Surely one of the best novels I've ever read'
Andrew Sean Greer, author of *Less*

'*Separate Rooms* is a stunning novel . . . If you ever need reminding why we run towards connection, even in the face of risk and loss, read this book, and prepare to be deeply moved'
Jack Parlett, author of *Fire Island*

'A major work of queer literature . . . Bleak and harrowingly funny and eventually gloriously redemptive'
Will Tosh, author of *Straight Acting*

'A discreet, lyrical meditation on the nature of male love'
Edmund White

Pier Vittorio Tondelli was born in Correggio in 1955 and died in 1991. He made his debut in 1980 with *Altri libertini*, which was followed in 1982 by *Pao Pao*. In 1985 he published the novel *Rimini*, followed by *Biglietti agli amici* in 1986 and *Separate Rooms* in 1989.

Separate Rooms

Pier Vittorio Tondelli

Translated by Simon Pleasance

With an introduction by André Aciman

Sceptre

Original title: CAMERE SEPARATE
© 2017 Giunti Editore S.p.A. / Bompiani, Firenze-Milano
1989 First publication under Bompiani imprint
2017 First publication as Bompiani / Giunti Editore S.p.A.
First published in Great Britain in 1992 by Serpent's Tail, London

This edition first published in 2025 by Sceptre
An imprint of Hodder & Stoughton Limited
An Hachette UK company

The authorised representative in the EEA is Hachette Ireland,
8 Castlecourt Centre, Castleknock Road, Castleknock, Dublin
15, D15 XTP3, Republic of Ireland (email: info@hbgi.ie)

2

Copyright © Pier Vittorio Tondelli 1989
English translation © Simon Pleasance 1992
Introduction © André Aciman 2025

The right of Pier Vittorio Tondelli to be identified as the
Author of the Work has been asserted by him in accordance
with the Copyright, Designs and Patents Act 1988.

A CIP catalogue record for this title is available from the British Library

Hardback ISBN 9781399734493
Trade Paperback ISBN 9781399734509
ebook ISBN 9781399734523

Typeset in Sabon MT by Hewer Text UK Ltd, Edinburgh
Printed and bound in Great Britain by Clays Ltd, Elcograf S.p.A.

Hodder & Stoughton policy is to use papers that are natural, renewable
and recyclable products and made from wood grown in sustainable
forests. The logging and manufacturing processes are expected to
conform to the environmental regulations of the country of origin.

Hodder & Stoughton Limited
Carmelite House
50 Victoria Embankment
London EC4Y 0DZ

www.sceptrebooks.co.uk

Contents

INTRODUCTION

André Aciman

Soon after leaving Cambridge in my very early thirties, I realised how much I missed the friends I'd left behind there. Once I was settled in New York, I began writing to each one. Those were the days before email existed, so all I had outside of costly long-distance phone calls was writing letters – long, fastidiously elaborate letters where I related incidents and feelings that, in normal day-to-day conversations, I might have been reluctant to share. On paper, though, I found myself opening up with unsparing abandon, shamelessly writing how much their friendship had meant to me and how I missed our walks at night when we'd put aside our books to roam from bar to bar. To others, I wrote how I missed Sunday afternoons that could so easily morph into evenings as we drank wines of choice vintage before realising that dinner would never materialise unless someone started to cook something. I loved these friends who never left Cambridge and kept summoning me back to a rhythm of life that seemed far more amenable than New York's rugged wake-up call.

My letters to them were effusive. I missed them. That was undeniable. But there were moments when, after signing my name and licking the envelope, a doubt would surge and make me wonder whether I'd been entirely sincere with them. Was I as homesick for Cambridge as I claimed to be? Were my yearnings the result of having moved to a city where I didn't know a soul? Or, as I grew to suspect, did the act of writing and telling them how much I missed our bars and their gardens make me more nostalgic than I really was? In other words, did reminiscing cast a luminous aura that existed less in reality than in the lime-lit, cadenced sentences I put to paper?

Language is always rhetorical – even when it doesn't mean to be.

It is perhaps because of this, and after reading Mattia Mossali's doctoral dissertation devoted in good part to the novel, that I instantly responded to Pier Vittorio Tondelli's *Separate Rooms*.

The story is about a visceral and indomitable attraction between two men – Leo is an Italian writer and thirty-two years old; Thomas, a pianist, is German and significantly younger – that soon enough morphs into a very powerful love. But one sentence in particular stood out and told me that I was in the hands, not of an occasional writer, but of one who had fathomed both himself and his true, complex, frequently unsortable emotions. His capacity to probe and articulate these contradictory strains arrested me and presaged a writer never pleased with easy answers. In that momentous sentence, Thomas knows he is Leo's lifelong partner; but he feels stuck on the margins of their relationship each time Leo disappears, or needs to travel on a journalistic assignment, or retreats into his brooding, solitary life. 'You want to keep me at a safe distance so you can write to me,' he says. 'If I lived with you . . . you wouldn't be able to think of me like a character in your stage production' (196). This was indeed the case with my friends in Cambridge. I needed them at a safe distance to convey my love for them. Nearby, speech would have served the purpose easily enough. But writing involved something far more complicated. Writing feeds on distance, but it could just as easily breed that distance. Writing, as I was finding out, is never about the obvious; it needs to excavate the obvious and give it new words.

Which is why Leo needs his privacy, his solitude, his space. Leo loves Thomas, but he cannot live with him. In Leo's own words, theirs is 'a relationship . . . that involved belonging to each other, but not possessing each other' (187). This in effect spells the reason for the novel's title, *Separate Rooms*.

This is not how Leo and Thomas's relationship begins. It starts quite quickly when, after running into Thomas at a party in Paris and getting to know him slightly better at another party, also set in Paris, the two grow aware of their instant attraction, what with 'their disguised nonchalant contact, [their] light skimming touches, and . . . silent glances' (17). They haven't spoken a word to each other, but they already know.

The two agree to meet at a rock concert. At first Leo has difficulty spotting Thomas in the crowd but eventually he finds him, and their connection is instantaneous. Their love, as Tondelli notes, is simply *epic*. They travel a great deal together, and Leo is constantly flying around the globe, but he always returns to seek out Thomas, and Thomas is always ready to welcome him.

All Leo needs – to use my word again – is space.

The point can't be made clearer when immediately after leaving by train one day, a bereft Thomas suddenly materialises and buzzes downstairs at Leo's building. 'I want to stay here and live with you,' he says once Leo lets him in. To this Leo replies, 'So you've decided to live in Italy?' (181).

Thomas did not come to live in Italy. He came to live with Leo. And Leo knows it.

Eventually the two quarrel, as they frequently have in the past. But, as Tondelli writes, 'They always ended up getting back together again' (62). Thomas leaves Leo's apartment. On the landing, as he waits for the elevator to arrive, he hears Leo shut and bolt the door behind him.

One might expect this to be a clean break. But it is not. Their love is limitless, though love, even when perfect, remains a dysfunctional bargain.

The problem with them is not only that Leo wants them to have their proverbial separate rooms, where Leo can 'go on being a separate lover . . . [and dream] his love, and . . . not . . . get stuck in everyday life.' The problem is that 'if they lived together, they would become caricatures of each other, like two obscene, face-lifted twins in a Berlin cabaret' (183).

What Leo can't grapple with – and here it's important to keep in mind that the novel was published in 1989 and therefore written in the late eighties – is that there existed a highly undefined template for a gay life. Leo 'had no models to follow, no experience to recycle and fall back on in this stage of their relationship. He knew that the love he still felt for Thomas would not be enough on its own. They would tear each other to pieces and that was the last thing he wanted . . . Living together meant believing in values that neither of them was capable of recognising. How would their love end?' (182)

This is why Tondelli's novel, as much as it spoke to its readership in the early nineties, was also proposing a sort of relationship that the gay community might have regarded as highly unusual. For though there is no doubting their love and desire for each other, Leo and Thomas didn't live together. And Tondelli not only resists established norms for gay couples but goes further yet to make light of 'normalised' gay couples:

Would they have no option but to normalise a relationship that society was in fact incapable of accepting as something normal? Would they not turn into the mirror image of those grotesque homosexual couples where one does all the cooking and the other always goes to the market to do the shopping? Where the two lovers resemble each other in their attitudes, in their way of doing things, even in their facial expressions, to the point where they become two pathetic replicas of one and the same unbearable imaginary male, emasculated and effeminate? In the

course of time would they not become two hysterical androids, forever on the point of butting in every
time the other spoke, with that facial skin that is a
bit too smooth and taut and tanned, and that hair
that is a bit too perfect the way it hides thinning
spots? (182)

What Leo wants is entirely different. He wants intimacy,
both physical and emotional, but he needs space. Can the
world adjust to this? Can Thomas? Can Leo even?

One day, Thomas announces he is seeing a woman
called Susann. This throws Leo completely off. His relationship with Thomas is hardly threatened by Susann,
yet he resents her intrusion into their lives. What Leo
leaves out of this equation is that his relationship with
Thomas is itself already riddled by his need for privacy
and solitude. Susann fills a void that was already partially
empty.

At the start of the novel, Thomas dies.

This leaves Leo not only grief-stricken, but totally
rudderless and unable to move forward. In fact, there is
no forward anything. Another relationship after Thomas
is simply unthinkable. Leo's hollowed out existence
becomes his new mode of living. Friends criticise him,
some even remind Leo that Thomas was just an insignificant somebody he hooked up with at a party in Paris but
rarely spent much time with, and who was vowed to fail
as a musician. Leo needs a wake-up call.

But Leo does not find another lover. He resurrects old
friendships he might have unintentionally discarded or

neglected. Eventually he forges newer ones, but the novel is a scatter of recollections of Thomas. Leo traipses around the world either seeking or escaping experiences he is unable to name or fathom. But then he'll recall travels with Thomas that brought him so much joy and love. These belong to the past now.

The wake-up call his friends want him to heed never comes.

Until it does come, in an oblique, quiet, almost incidental manner. It's a call that has been summoning him for ever so long, both from recollections of Thomas but also from deep within himself, going back to his earliest childhood. It has to do with his ability to say 'in words what others are quite happy to remain silent about' (226). It also explains the genius of *Separate Rooms*. For it's a novel both exceptionally moving yet exceptionally lucid as it weaves its way through the twisted strands of what Leo is desperately trying to unearth and parse in himself.

And this is when it hits him in the face. The reason for needing separate rooms couldn't be simpler. Leo has always been cut off from the world around him because, unlike everyone else, he is a writer. Because he is different. 'He has roots in no town. He has no family or children. He does not have a house that you could really call "home".' More importantly, his sexuality underscores that difference: 'What he lacks most of all is a companion. He is single, and alone' (3). Tondelli writes: 'If he did not manage to function with Thomas, if his emotional life is a mess, if, deep down, he is restless and will never find peace, it is because he is different, because he must construct a set of values that starts from the very fact that he is different' (226). His home is grounded on his ability to write about his and Thomas's love and about the loss of that love. For him, writing and love are indissolubly fused. It just took him a few years after Thomas to see this.

What is truly sad is that Tondelli himself was to die on 16 December 1991, of complications related to AIDS. He was thirty-six years old.

My life in New York was not troubled by the death of a dear one, but I had lost people who were very dear to me and who were, as I knew they would be, irreplaceable. Years later the two souls who had invited me to their garden so many times on those glorious Sunday afternoons to drink Château Beychevelle and Château Cos d'Estournel with them did die two ignominious deaths: she in a fire that burned down their home; he in a hospital bed, while everyone who cherished him waited for news, knowing that the longer he stayed in a coma, the slimmer his chances. I never said farewell to either. But then I'd been saying farewell to them for years – though I never suspected they'd ever actually be gone from my life, the way Leo never believed Thomas would leave his. With the friends who died I might have been overstating my attachment to them and, perhaps, I was stylising how much I missed them, but I also knew that what writing made me say was more deliberate, more genuine, more heartfelt, and ultimately more enjoyable than what I might have said in a rushed phone call from New York.

In some instances, what one loves are not just people or

places but the act of writing about our love for them. Writing finds love and stirs it when it is all but gone everywhere else. I was writing from love and with love, already sensing that when someone is gone from our life, all we are left with are words.

New York, 2024

Separate Rooms

FIRST MOVEMENT

Into Silence

One day, not so very long ago, he caught himself looking at his face mirrored in the window of a small plane flying from Paris to Munich.

Twenty-five thousand feet below, the Alps looked like ripples of sand, tinged with gold by the setting sun. The deep blue sky seemed fathomless, lit on the horizon by a bright saffron hem, the colour of Zen robes.

The landscape framed in the small oval window conjured up night and day, and the boundaries between two worlds: earth and air. Later, when a light went on in the cabin, reflecting his weary, fuller face on that northerly holographic screen, the landscape told him things about himself as well.

His face, the one which others had for years recognised as 'his', once again struck him as foreign. Every day his face seemed more alien, because the image he retained of his own face was forever and eternally his face as a boy and as a younger man.

1

He still thought of himself and saw himself as an innocent, someone incapable of doing ill or going astray. But
the image he saw against that illuminated backdrop was
simply the face of someone no longer as young as he used
to be: someone with fine, thinning hair, puffy eyes, full
and slightly flabby lips, and the skin of the cheeks flecked
with fine veins, just like his father's livid cheeks. All in all
a face suffering, like any other, the deterioration and the
marks of time.

He turned thirty-two just a few months back. He is
well aware that he is not of an age ordinarily defined as
mature or, even less, old. But he also knows that he is not
young any more. Most of his university friends have
married and had children. Most of them own a home and
have a fairly well paid profession. When he bumps into
them, on those rare visits to his parents' home – the house
he was born in, and later fled from on the pretext of
pursuing his studies – he senses that there is an ever deep-
ening gulf between himself and them. His old friends pay
taxes, just like he does. They take summer holidays and
have to insure the car, just like he does. But on the odd
occasion when they get to talking, he realises that they
have altogether different responsibilities. He realises that
in their respective lives they have roles that have absolutely nothing in common. As a result he feels more and
more alone, or rather, more and more aloof and different. He has broken away from the surroundings where he
grew up, and lives each day detached from the comforting
day-to-day life of a small community. He has time on his
hands that others do not have. This in itself makes him
different. He is pursuing an artistic profession, but here,

too, he has little in common with his so-called colleagues. This makes him feel all the more different. He has roots in no town. He has no family or children. He does not have a house that you could really call 'home'. Yet another difference. But what he lacks most of all is a companion. He is single, and alone.

The plane suddenly loses altitude as it starts its descent towards Munich. He turns away from the window and gathers up his things. He puts away the book he had been leafing through, slips his glasses into their case, and puts out his cigarette. He leans his head back. They will be touching down in twenty minutes or so. He imagines Thomas pacing nervously back and forth in the international arrivals hall, checking his watch and the scheduled landing times. He sees his lanky form heading impatiently towards a row of shop-windows with displays of pipe tobacco and gaudy boxes of Havana cigars. He imagines his frayed sweater, his thick woollen jacket, his velvet trousers, his big, stout, red leather shoes. He sees the dark pools of his eyes, his broad, relaxed smile, his warm, bony arms that will hug him as they always do and steer him firmly to a beat-up Citroën or Renault, parked miles away. But he cannot hear his voice. He sees their embrace quite clearly, he picks up the sweet smell of his skin, he feels his cheek rough with its two-day growth, he sees his lips asking softly 'How was your trip?', but he cannot hear the sound or inflexion of that voice. He sees their embrace, but he cannot feel it.

He heaves a sigh, eyes closed, head still tipped against the lowered back of the seat. The stewardess leans over and says a few words to him. Slowly he emerges from his reverie and adjusts the back of his seat to the upright position, ready for landing. His eyes are open again now. With an inner shudder of horror, he is once more fully aware of what is tritely called reality, though he prefers to call it 'the current state of this dream'. There will be no Thomas waiting to meet him at the airport with his dilapidated Citroën. Nor will there be any friend in his place. Because Thomas, or at least everything on this earth that bore this name and everything that had anything to do with this name, for himself and for those who loved him, Thomas is no more. Thomas is dead. Two years now. And he feels more and more alone. More alone and even more different.

A few years back, on the sort of grim, grey Sunday that only the skies of Northern Europe can come up with, Leo left a brasserie in Paris with Michael, an American jazz musician. Michael, if the truth be told, was just another of those expatriates who turn up in farflung corners of the world as a result of discontent or restlessness.

Michael is a man of forty, heavily built, with a full beard turning white on his chin. He is more bald than not, with a face that might be best likened to a potato field – full of growths, pimples and lumps. He usually wears military trousers held up by black leather braces, woollen shirts, and a black felt hat, Rainer Fassbinder-style. He chews on all kinds of cigars, especially when he gets involved in all-night jam sessions. By dawn, he is invariably the only member of the band still on his feet. Leo likes Michael. He likes the music he plays, too. He would never dream of talking about literature or philosophy with him, but they find plenty to say about Broadway music shows. And young men. One of those Sunday afternoons that seem so long ago, Michael and Leo left a brasserie in the Marais to go to a party. Leo met Thomas at that party. Or rather, Leo saw Thomas for the first time.

They walk side by side through the Place des Vosges, staring at the ground and talking as if they were addressing the cobblestone pavement. Both have their hands thrust deep in their pockets and their necks wrapped in long scarves. The November chill is like dry, invisible snow melted in the air. They reach the building where the party is. They can hear music and hubbub wafting down into the street. Other party-goers run past and reach the doorway ahead of them. Leo smiles and slips his arm through Michael's. They climb to the fourth floor. They have to avoid stepping on people who have spilled out on to the landing and stairway. Empty champagne bottles are rolling about on the wooden floorboards covered with confetti and cigarette butts. Inside there is crush and confusion, people dancing, people smoking dope, people drinking whisky straight from the bottle. Leo pulls Michael over to the drinks table. A young punk girl with a plume of iridescent hair dazzles him taking flash photos with her polaroid. Further in, images of the party fill the TV screens scattered around the apartment. Some young men are filming the party with a video camera. They push through the throng, spotlighting the guests like some night-fishing expedition: in the beam of the powerful light, small darting fish, confident and quick, suddenly turn phosphorescent, as do handsome lobsters – elderly and inebriated, sharks, pink prawns, garish tropical fish, whales, dolphins and the odd bream. Leo steps back out of their way. He says hello to various people he knows, with kisses, hugs and handshakes. Then he finally reaches the room where the food is. Two round tables littered with torn paper plates and napkins, ashtrays overflowing with cigarette stubs, and leftovers. Beyond the tables, the drinks. He pours himself a glass of champagne, then another and a third, to get himself into the swing of things. The wild disco music has a vaguely African beat. Everyone is moving. Leo sways, uncorks another bottle and offers Michael a drink.

'Leo, Leo!' shouts the host, edging his way towards him, hands high above the heads of the crowd. He is dressed up like a geisha. 'My dear, thanks for coming! Some party, isn't it? We've been at it since last night. I showed the movie, you know. It was a great hit!'

Leo hugs Bernard and compliments him on his fiery red kimono. He introduces Michael to him. He makes small talk for a moment or two, until Bernard is whisked off by other friends, all singing his praises, and shouting his name. Someone thrusts the camera into his hand. Bernard climbs on to a table, looks through the view-finder and pretends to shoot Leo. Everybody cheers. Leo giggles. Bernard yells something, then passes the camera to someone else and disappears, engulfed by the crush of admirers. 'Let's have a look at the crazy old queen's film,' Leo says to Michael after a while.

In the throng, they elbow their way through Bernard's apartment. Each room is a mixture of styles: papier mâché columns, Second Empire mirrors and pier glasses, here and there a Bauhaus armchair, a Renaissance confessional fitted with bookshelves, rugs, damask hangings, tapestries, spray-painted Moorish cupolas made of poly-styrene, rejects and remains from all Bernard's past sets: reminders of his irrepressible kitsch style and his dream-like zaniness. White statues of demigods sporting gigan-tic copper-coloured phalluses; capitals and columns; coloured plaster of Paris figures of St Sebastian, implor-ing or sublimely absent in the hour of his martyrdom; in the windows, figures of Mary Magdalene, Christ on the cross, Angels and Archangels, and Thrones. They pass through four reception rooms until the chattering, tipsy party fauna thins out. They still have to cross the exercise room and the bathroom before they eventually reach Bernard's large bedroom where his latest video is being shown on multiple screens.

In this room people are sprawled on rugs and the bed, some asleep in front of the screen. Leo and Michael lean against a corner of the four-poster bed and watch the video. After a while Michael leaves in search of more alcohol.

It is just at that moment that Leo becomes aware of someone brushing past him. From his slightly precarious position against the spiral bedpost, all he catches is a glimpse of someone's legs passing the mirror on the door – just jeans and a pair of black shoes. But an irresistible urge makes him get to his feet. He leaves the bedroom, following the young man with his gaze. He stops in his tracks momentarily, not sure whether to keep up his pursuit or go back and watch the video. Then Michael comes back, saying he has found a horn to play. Making their way through the guests they reach a dimly lit room filled with smoke. Somebody is playing the piano. Michael

7

picks up an old sax and starts to blow. Leo's eyes linger softly on the young man at the piano. He examines him intently. He is seeing Thomas for the first time. And as if Thomas can feel the charge of Leo's gaze, he raises his head and stares back for a split second. Then his eyes return just as fast to the keyboard and he starts rocking to and fro, in time to Michael's rhythm. Leo refills his glass.

Some time later Leo is slumped in an enormous damasked armchair, answering a Spanish journalist's questions in that overly polite manner that tipsiness sometimes brings out in him. He sees Thomas leaving the apartment with a girl. He feels like getting up and following him. He braces his legs, gripping the arms of the chair. But his strength fails him and he topples heavily backwards. The journalist asks him if he's writing anything at the moment. A smile flickers across Leo's face and he carries on chatting about this and that.

A few evenings later Rodolfo phones from Milan. He asks how things are going in Paris, if the apartment is all right, and if there is anything he can do for him. Leo answers a little testily. He has known Rodolfo for the best part of ten years. They are the same age. They know more or less everything there is to know about each other's lives. It was Rodolfo who found Leo a place to live in Paris. Rodolfo is a handsome man about to turn thirty. He is an architect, specialising in 1950s decor. He has designed select bars from Milan to Florence, and earned quite a name for himself. He contributes to an international furniture magazine. He combines the necessary worldliness with intelligence and a sense of irony. He loves Leo, as one might love one's own gay brother.

'I'm getting the hang of things,' Leo replies. 'Don't worry yourself. I'm seeing Michael. I told you about him, didn't I? I get about, and I sleep . . .' He is already keen to get off the phone, fill his glass with ice and drown it with rum. Rodolfo picks up on this kind of mood. So he slowly lets slip the only topic that might keep Leo on the line. 'I saw Hermann the other night. He's getting on fine, you know.'

Leo leans close to the mouthpiece: 'Hermann?'

'He's living fifteen miles north of Rome. He asked me for your address. I pretended I didn't know it. We were in a bar . . . I was on the point of giving it to him. Then I thought I'd better ask you first.'

Leo sighs. 'You did the right thing. Ever since we split up—'

'I just wanted to tell you he seems to be doing fine,' Rodolfo interrupts. 'His work's going well. He's having a show or two. Nothing big, but for him . . . I think it's important, don't you?'

'I'm glad you called first,' Leo repeats frostily.

'I couldn't make up my mind . . . You were both so happy together, I mean . . . Believe me, Leo, I really don't want to interfere in your love life, but I thought you should know he asked me about you, and I'm sure he meant it.'

'I met someone the other night,' Leo says quietly.

Rodolfo's voice stiffens: 'Are you serious?'

'It's all over with Hermann. I wouldn't be here if there'd been the slightest chance of getting back together. I'll probably always love him. He knows it, too. But I want to get away from him. Only a lunatic would try to get a divorced couple back together again. A lot of people just won't understand. But it's just the same for two men.'

'Unless one of the two queens goes by the name of Liz Taylor,' Rodolfo adds.

Silence for a moment, then a burst of laughter. Leo loves Rodolfo, loves him dearly.

'So what's with this new boy?' Rodolfo asks between guffaws. 'Another Chez Maxim's? No, no . . . I hope he's not a "wrong blonde". Everybody hopes that, after Hermann. Or maybe he's . . . Leo, don't tell me you've found . . .'

Leo says nothing. He would rather arouse Rodolfo's curiosity. Rodolfo has never committed himself to anyone and may be totally incapable of being in love. He likes people courting him, and he often switches partners. He reckons there's something pathetic about two men living together: one of them invariably ends up being like a housemaid. Rodolfo lives quite happily with his filofax packed with addresses from all round the world.

'Don't tell me you've found a Vondel Park! That would be too much!'

'I haven't talked to him yet. You know how I am in this sort of situation. You'd have ended up in bed already.'

'Leo, I'm just hoping he's not a Whitman. You're in Paris to get yourself back together a bit, and what d'you go and do? Fall for a Whitman.'

'I can't tell you anything more for now,' Leo rejoins laughing.

'But have you found out where he lives? Why not throw a little party in your place. Invite him along. Maybe I'll pop up to Paris to give you a hand.'

Leo straightaway changes the subject. Then he says his goodbyes to Rodolfo. He does not ask anything about Hermann. He hangs up the receiver, goes to the kitchen, and fills a glass with ice. He looks at his collection of favourite rums: a Barbancourt five star, a Myers's, a nameless Venezuelan rum, an Indian Old Monk. He chooses the right one for the occasion: the Haitian. It is lighter and at the same time more perfumed. His passion for rum is possibly the only passion he ever managed to pass on to Hermann.

The Parisian sky appears in the pane of the bathroom window. The other rooms look out on to an inner court-yard. Leo sits on the edge of the bathtub and thinks of Thomas. Thomas is definitely not a Chez Maxim's. At first sight, he does not look like everybody's ideal man, the sort of person who welcomes the world with open arms, without taking a close look first, and testing the water. As Christopher Isherwood would put it, people who go to Chez Maxim's are already fair game. If it's Chez Maxim's, it's the best. People do not bother to ask if it is really any good. You see some rugged, suntanned man, well-built, with chiselled features, his body bristling with muscles. All of a sudden you are identifying with your own dream ticket; you are saying how fabulous everything is – here is the man of my life, the one and only. But things are not like that. The meeting is just a symbol, and when all is said and done it has no meaning at all. People just keep on looking for Chez Maxim's – even in Anatolia when it would be a lot easier to have a quick picnic with goat's cheese and lettuce. This is the Chez Maxim's type. But Thomas has an inner quality, a way of looking that definitely gives people an impression that there is more to come.

He is probably not a Whitman either, Leo thinks to himself. Not the way Allen Ginsberg defined it. When Ginsberg reflected about his own partners and related them to previous relationships, he said he could copulate his way right back to Walt Whitman's lover as if making his way back through a noble family tree. The Whitman type is very common in the gay ghetto. If you scratch the surface a little you soon find out that they have all been to bed with everybody. Ginsberg adopts the theory that there is just one sodomite embrace: universal and parallel to Adam and Eve's. But for Leo, Thomas is neither a Chez Maxim's nor, from what he can tell right now, a Whitman.

He is not a 'wrong blonde' either – the definition that Wystan Auden gave to Chester Kallmann, who became his lifelong companion. The story goes that just after Auden arrived in the United States, he was infatuated by a fair-haired student at Brooklyn College called Walter Miller. He met him after a poetry reading at the League of American Writers. Miller was writing for the *Observer*, the College literary review. Chester, then eighteen, was the editor. So Auden arranged an appointment with Chester, quite sure that he would turn up for the interview with Miller in tow. When the blonde-haired Chester turned up alone on the doorstep, Auden went into the other room and whispered to Isherwood, who was sharing the apartment: 'It's the wrong blonde.'

Within a matter of hours, if we are to believe the biographers, Chester Kallmann became 'the only possible blonde' for Auden. Thomas is not a wrong blonde, in other words, not the only possible blonde. That person in Leo's life was definitely Hermann. Besides, Thomas does not have blonde hair.

Maybe he is more a Vondel Park. Physically, in fact, something of the Nordic type of the seventies lives on in him. A physical throwback that has nothing to do with what is worn, that is not imitated by fashions or reflected in clothes. Rather, it immediately summons up soul and background. Unlike the Chez Maxim's, you would never find a Vondel in fashion magazines. The Vondel always has an elusive quality, something slightly contaminated and worn, a whiff of dilapidation. Just to give an example: fingertips blackened from rolling cigarettes.

So what type is Thomas? Leo goes back to the kitchen. He pours himself another tumblerful of rum. He goes to the bedroom, puts on some music and undresses. Thomas is nobody, Leo says to himself, right now Thomas is absolutely nobody.

Leo's apartment is full of light and people now. There are never enough glasses, even though he and Michael have been at the sink washing dirty ones for a good half-hour. The smoked salmon is almost gone. The Lorum trout vanished in seconds. There are still a couple of platters of charcuterie left, some pears with Camembert and walnuts, and some cheese puffs. In the kitchen Thomas is opening a case of Bordeaux with a serrated knife. Leo is drying glasses and eyeing Thomas bent over the box. The atmosphere smacks of manly, domestic intimacy. Leo finds it pleasing. It gives him a sense of satisfaction. Every two or three minutes someone comes into the kitchen asking for a glass, or a plate, or a clean ashtray, or a bottle of Sancerre. Instead of saying anything, the three of them just snicker. The intruder realises that he could spend an hour asking the three gents to lend an ear, and still no one would help. He leaves thwarted, which prompts other remarks from them.

Michael has brought half a dozen guests along to the party, among them a *Women's Journal* correspondent, a sculptress from New Zealand on a scholarship to the Ecole des Beaux-Arts, a couple of musicians from his band, and Thomas, of course, invited deliberately for Leo. Those few hours they spent together jamming at Bernard's party serve as a letter of introduction. Leo, for his part, has invited people from the Parisian publishing scene, a few Italian journalists whom he is on good terms with, and an Argentine writer who lives in the neighbourhood. These are the people Leo knows, or who have been introduced to him. The rest of the human fauna filling his apartment, including the duty guests, is a hotchpotch, like so many bits of candied fruit in the icing on a cake. Leo does not know who they are. The party started at nine. Between nine and ten all he did was answer the doorbell, shake hands, and throw in a few polite words in three or four languages. A little later, as soon as he realised that the party had taken off and could happily carry on under its own steam, he disappeared into the kitchen to wash glasses and smoke a cigarette in peace. Thomas was at the piano again. Leo brushed against his back and gave him a thank-you-for-coming smile. No words passed between them. Not long after, Michael brought Thomas into the kitchen. And now, with a chuckle every so often, they were quietly together, in perfect unison.

14

Leo can sense Thomas's presence, close to, like an aura of tenderness which he wants to be part of at the earliest opportunity. He feels like caressing Thomas's face and holding him tightly in his arms. He has nothing to say to him, though he feels that Thomas has already started to get to know him. When Leo makes a quip at Michael, he senses that Thomas understands. He knows that Thomas is watching him. Here and now he is not quite sure how the night will end, or what their next meeting might be like, but he knows that Thomas is right for him, and feels that he might become important for Thomas, too. Leo cannot tell how it all might turn out in the end. He has often wasted time pursuing someone who was not right for him. A tricky business. Wearisome phone-calls, meetings forever being put off, seduction strategies, making sure you are seen in certain places, train journeys, and meals with people with whom you would otherwise never ever have passed the time of day. Leo was younger then. He needed a partner, and he had to go looking for one. Then, one day, there was Hermann, and nothing was ever the same again.

Leo knows now that with this sort of thing you have to bide your time and be patient. You have to prepare yourself, and be aware that, in so doing, it will be easier to fall into step with the other person when he does appear. This is what is happening with Thomas. As soon as Leo saw him and felt his presence, he knew every part of him was involved. Even without Michael's help, he would have seen Thomas again somewhere. He knew that would not have been a problem. No one can keep two people apart when those two people belong to one another, when they have been seeking each other out, possibly for a very long time, and from a considerable distance.

Thomas is here, close to him, and for the time being this is all that matters. He feels that Thomas is showing him that he is available, even if rather naively and awkwardly – possibly even unawares. Thomas is still treating him superficially and casually. Leo will have to move things on to a deeper level. He will have to get closer to him, but discreetly, and show him that he is serious and interested. He will have to make Thomas understand that it may be his body and his intimacy that he passionately longs for at this moment, but he will also want his company if everything turns out right. He will want Thomas to become his friend. The partner to be with for the rest of his life.

Thomas is bent over the case of wine. Michael asks him if he is okay, if he needs a hand. Thomas answers with a snort: what's so difficult about opening a case of Bordeaux? Leo turns round from the sink and looks at him tenderly. They take the bottles from the box and set them on the white marble kitchen table, making sure that their bodies touch as they do so. Throughout the rest of the evening, whenever they happen to be close to one another, they brush hands, arms, shoulders and legs, but no one else is remotely aware of their contact. At one point, Leo lays a hand on Thomas's shoulder and asks him to make a path through the milling guests. Then Thomas puts a hand on Leo's hips, pushing him a little bit off course. As the party proceeds, so the two of them gradually create a language between their bodies, a code that nobody can yet decipher, because nobody knows the keyword: attraction. But things are stirring between Leo and Thomas, things are starting to move by the minute. The power behind it all lies in its very momentum. It comes from their disguised nonchalant contact, from those light skimming touches, and from those silent glances. They have not said a word to each other yet. There is no question of words being spoken in this shared moment that is so elemental and time-honoured. It is a moment when life summons life from the very depths of the species' energy. The sophistication of words would merely blur a moment that cannot be expressed by any language, except, perhaps, the language of life's struggle, implanted within the farthest recesses of the brain.

By about midnight there are only half a dozen people left. The duty guests are saying their goodbyes, and thanking Leo for his food and hospitality. Leo wanders downstairs with them to the street, where there is more handshaking. He waits in the doorway for the cars to drive off. He does this a couple of times. When at last he closes the apartment door behind him, panting a little from fatigue, he sees what a mess everything is. Tables covered with bottles, ashtrays brimful, scraps of food on plates piled high on shelves and windowsills and radiators. In a corner, the murmur of four guests drinking brandy. Someone is changing the music on the stereo. The records he has used for the party have not been put back in their sleeves. To his horror, Leo sees them heaped any old how in a corner, inviting dust and cigarette ash and spray from champagne.

Thomas is chatting with Michael in the other room. He suggests they pay a quick visit to Les Halles for a beer, and then maybe take in some music at the 'Baiser Salé'. Leo is game, but he wants ten minutes to get ready. He goes to his bedroom and flings himself on to the bed. His arm reaches out to the bedside table and his fingertips search for his box of hashish. He picks it up, opens it, chooses a little lump and fills a pipe. He wants to be alone with that young man. He wonders if tonight will be the right night. It depends on him, on his energy, and how well he seduces him. It depends on how available Thomas is. Too many things. Better to let everything drift, like the smoke that is starting to take effect, filling out his lungs like an ethereal, euphoric hit of being high.

The following evening Leo calls Thomas at home. A girl answers, and asks him to hang on for a moment. Leo starts circling the table in his study, telephone in hand. Eventually he recognises Thomas's voice. When they have said their hellos, Thomas tells him how the night ended, and Leo apologises for dropping off to sleep. But there is something odd about the tone of Thomas's voice and possibly about the pauses in his version of things, too. Neither of them is averse to resorting to polite clichés, for they are not familiar enough yet to have an unadorned conversation. They are two people in search of each other, two individuals who still do not really know anything about one another, apart from the visible aspects of their personalities, or the kind of details you find in any pass-port: height, profession, place of birth, and age.

'I'd like to have an evening just with you,' Leo says in the end, lowering his voice. 'We could go to the theatre, or a movie . . .'

'When?'

'Tonight if you're free.'

Thomas stalls. 'There's a concert at the Zenith next Friday. I'm going with a few friends. We could meet there.'

Leo is not thrilled at the idea. He did say '. . . an evening just with you', and here is Thomas proposing a package tour. He does not answer.

'See you on Friday then?' Thomas asks, insistent.

'I'm really not sure,' Leo blurts out. He does not like it when things don't turn out the way he has planned.

Thomas realises what is going on. 'I want to see you too,' he says softly. 'Try and make it on Friday.'

The night of the concert Leo gets to the Zenith late. He took too long buying drugs from a dealer at the café where he hangs out. He bought five grammes of marijuana in a small packet that is now flattened in the inside pocket of his jacket. He wants to try some right away. In mid-street he fills the bowl of his pipe, hardly slowing his pace as he does so. It's good dope, perhaps just a little too sweet. Best to add another twist of tobacco.

By the time he reaches the auditorium, the group has already played a couple of numbers. He recognises the start of a song, which is met by a roar. A shower of pink carnations pours down on to the audience from the middle of the roof. The singer comes on stage with a 'Bonsoir Paris.' The stage lights flash on and off, dozens and dozens of flashes in every colour imaginable: pastel pink, pale green, light blue, orange, flame red, yellow, and finally climaxing with the blinding white of the arc lights.

Leo is feeling euphoric. His legs are shaking a little from running to the show, from the loud shrieking all around him, and from the fact of being plunged into a crowd, something which always gives him an immediate feeling of suffocating, be it in a concert stadium or a sports arena. Then it all passes, as long as he realises that he himself is no longer merely a lone individual, but part of a collective whole. So he starts looking at the show with the crowd's eyes rather than his own. He lets the music take him over, abandoning himself to the gyrations of the people around him – a sea of fair hair and very young faces, dancing, pushing and screaming. The boom of the music is deafening. Several thousand people packed into the hall, sweating, smoking, shouting, dancing, kissing and hugging, tossing clothes into the air, jostling with each other to get close to the stage, way over there. Leo sticks to the edge of the crowd, by a makeshift stand where they are selling bottles of beer. He tries to get his bearings, and looks upwards scanning the two balconies bursting with fans. He will never find Thomas. It would be a miracle, even though he has always sincerely believed in miracles. He downs one beer after another until he really feels part of the collective surge, singing and dancing. He sways with the music, lights a cigarette and shakes his head. The band plays on for a good half-hour. Then during a frenzied drum solo a spotlight starts to zigzag through the audience, capturing it in a narrow, dazzling cone of light. Leo suddenly switches off from the music and follows the pool of light straying among the heads of the spectators, winding between the pillars in the auditorium, lingering on the roof, and then lighting up the crowd below like a spotter plane. And as Leo follows the light he suddenly spots Thomas.

He sees him for a split second up in the balcony to the left, close to the stage, sitting on the floor with his feet dangling in space. He is not shouting. He is almost motionless, except for his legs swinging to and fro. His head is resting on his arms crossed on the railing, like a small boy absent-mindedly watching a film. Leo feels a surge of tenderness rise up within him. He tries to join Thomas. He leaves the hall and climbs the stairway leading to the balconies. But when he finds himself up against a solid wall of people, on the other side of the doors, he realises he will never reach Thomas this way. He goes back down to the auditorium. He wants to attract Thomas's attention. Make a rendezvous, at least in sign language, outside the theatre so that they will not both get lost in the crowd. So he starts pushing past people, squeezing his way through groups of fans, kicking over cans of beer, rubbing against sweating shoulders and backs, slowly edging his way inch by inch to the middle of the auditorium. He moves as if he is in a maze, a few steps in one direction, a few feet further in another, then back on his tracks again, endlessly shifting course. He makes the most of the invisible spaces between people. When he feels he has reached a dead end, he thrusts his way forward again. Now and then he looks up. Thomas is still there, not more than twenty yards away, but impossible to reach.

The music drives to a crescendo. The electronic drumbeats pounding out several thousand watts make the whole dome vibrate. The lighting onstage is bright red. The spectators twist and writhe, turning this way and that, swaying in fits and starts, but in perfect time to the

music. People are jumping up and down, others are shouting, frenzied heads of hair shaking, arms stretching
upward, long and straight, black curly hair, necks dripping with sweat, backs and legs and chests all shaking
and moving. Leo suddenly finds himself in the middle of
a group of five or six fans dancing in a circle, defending
their space like wild animals. They have thrown their
jackets, coats, bags, pullovers and scarves into a heap on
the floor. The girls in the group come all round him laughing, pushing him and bumping him with quick flicks of
their hips, luring him into their dance. Leo smiles and
yells something. A girl throws her arms round him and
kisses him, trying to pull him closer to her. Leo manages
to escape her clutches and makes headway until he is right
underneath the balcony. He starts to call Thomas's name,
waving his arms and gesticulating to catch his eye. But to
no avail. The music suddenly stops. The lights go out,
leaving just the rotating sphere of mirrors bouncing its
reflections round and round the walls of the auditorium
and over the bodies of the fans. The concert is over. The
crowd whistles, shrieks and shouts. People call for an
encore. Leo keeps calling out to Thomas, but in vain. All
of a sudden a different rhythm starts to fill the large hall.
At first it is quite faint, then it becomes clearer and more
insistent. It comes from the back of the hall, from the
gods and the balconies, and floods across the auditorium.
The rumble gradually smothers all the shouts and shrieks,
the whistles and applause. They are stamping on the
wooden floor, ten to start with, then fifty and a hundred,
and now two thousand. The atmosphere is surreal, as if a
primitive tribe had started a war dance. No voices or

shouting, but serious, tense faces, clenched jaws and closed fists. Just a wild, frenzied din. Then the echo of applause, as if borne on another surge. It sweeps over the crowd, staccato clapping louder and louder. And when the beat reaches its peak the whole concert-hall explodes in a roar. The stage lights flash on and off, once, twice, blinding through the smoke. The band comes back and starts playing a demented version of 'I Feel Love'.

Thomas's legs are dangling no more than ten or twelve feet above Leo's head. Leo gives them a furious glance. He stoops down, picks up a battered carnation, adjusts the petals a little and tosses it up to Thomas, calling out his name once more. But the carnation drops back down not far from him. Leo then goes back on his tracks a few feet, looking for the girl who kissed him a few minutes before. He grabs her arm and motions to her to climb on to his shoulders. The girl smiles happily. Leo gives her a flower and points up to Thomas. He bends down, hoists her, knees astride, on to his shoulders, and staggers towards the balcony. This tower-like thing advancing through the crowd excites the people nearby, and they start dancing around him. Leo tries to keep his strength up. He is sweating, but his main concern is trying to keep from being knocked over by the pushing and shoving of the people dancing all round him. After a few yards the crush is so thick that Leo can make headway by leaning into the people pressed close to him. They reach Thomas. The girl stretches out her arms and can almost touch him. Just a few inches more. There is only one thing for it. Leo braces his legs and jumps up. The girl touches Thomas's feet. At last he realises what is happening below. He leans over and sees Leo. The girl throws the flower to him before an exhausted Leo lowers her abruptly to the floor. 'I'm here!' Leo shouts waving his arms.

Thomas smiles. 'Wait there. I'm coming down!' he yells.

He gets up and makes his way along the balcony, weaving through the crowd. Down below, Leo tries to keep pace with him. But it is impossible. Thomas reaches the railing and gestures to Leo that he will never be able to get down to him before the concert is over. They are disappointed, but resigned. They try to fix a place to meet, but that is impossible, too. The light in the auditorium goes on and off: moments of pitch darkness, and moments of blinding light. Leo suddenly sees Thomas climbing over the railing. The flashing strobe lights stop him seeing clearly what Thomas is up to. Then he guesses that Thomas is trying to lower himself down. Holding on to a gaggle of arms, he swings out into space. People notice what is going on. They scream and shout and clap, and raise their arms as if waiting for an angel to drop from above. Leo stretches his arms out too. The music is deafening. The spotlight sweeping over the heads of the crowd suddenly focuses on the raised arms, the singing and dancing, the laughter and the cries of encouragement: stadium fever. Thomas stretches down towards the crowd. Leo can already grab hold of his shoes. But the people above are still holding him by the arms. Pulled both ways, Thomas looks like a puppet being tugged at by two rival gangs. His face glows with excitement and delight. He cannot stay like this for long. Leo keeps telling him to let himself go. Thomas finally launches himself into a sea of arms and hot bodies. A fearsome roar goes up, a cheer of delight, a cry of triumph from those who have won their trophy.

Leo throws himself at Thomas and tries to pull him to his feet.

'So good to see you!' he shouts, his lips pressing against Thomas's ear to make himself heard.

Thomas cannot believe his eyes. With an effort, grabbing hold of anything that comes to hand, he finally manages to get to his feet. Leo looks proudly at him and holds out his arms. Thomas folds into his embrace, and holds Leo tightly, resting his head on his shoulder. Leo strokes his hair. They are surrounded by a jostling crowd of people, congratulating them and pushing them this way and that. They stay locked together, clasping each other in that swaying sea of excited people. 'I Feel Love' plays on, the beat ever more insistent. Leo's lips seek out Thomas's mouth. Coloured smoke wafts up from the stage. And there, amid the jubilation that marks the end of the concert, amid the clapping, chanting, and whistling, amid the smoke encircling them and blocking them from view for a few moments, squeezing each other until it hurts, they have the first kiss of their life.

The crowd lingers on outside the concert hall. Groups of people are talking about the concert. Girls dash to and fro across the street to get an autograph from the lead singer. Thomas has already said his goodbyes to the friends he was with. Now he is with Leo, at a loss for words, bewildered, excited and weary.

'I'd like you to come to my place,' he says in the end, his voice cracking and shy. 'Come on. Please. Come back to my place.' Leo puts Thomas at ease, stroking his face and running his fingers through his hair. A bus speeds past, lighting their faces with its headlights. 'Okay,' says Leo, 'let's take a cab and get out of here.'

Thomas lives in Montmartre, on a dark, uphill street. He leads Leo past rundown buildings and they climb to the third floor. They walk into a spacious room, its ceiling decorated with ivory-coloured Art Nouveau stucco. There is a rose ornament in the middle of the ceiling with bare wires dangling from it. French windows take up one side of the room, with the bed facing them. On the wall opposite the door there is an upright piano set into a series of laden bookshelves, filled mainly with sheets of paper, scores, coloured boxes with papers sticking out of them, and some little furry animals. Thomas turns on a small bluish spotlight, closes the door, puts his arms round Leo, and invites him to lie down on the carpet near the radiator.

Countless times, ever since he decided to call it quits with Hermann, Leo had wondered what his next love affair would be like. In fact, his attempt to split up with Hermann had dragged on for eighteen months, what with the inevitable reconciliations, the passion that refused to die, and his own physical desire. What will the next love look like? What physical form will it take? Love, after all, is something unique, Leo thinks to himself. It includes Hermann, or the memory of him, as well as every experience that follows after him. Love is absolute. You cannot ordain it, speed it up, avoid it or steer it. Love is fullness, a total experience. This is why Leo was sure he would find love again. What he was not sure of was how. He could not predict the turn of events that would

26

introduce love to him again, its precise physiognomy. And now, as he lies close to Thomas's excited body, he recognises that love has once more entered his life.

Now love is a lean and long-legged body, its limbs still those of a teenager, soft and sinuous, and princely. Love is a long face with a strong, square jaw. Love is two bright, dark eyes, with a lock of dark honey-coloured hair falling across them every so often. Love is a special way of moving the hands or letting them hang down by the legs. Last but not least, love is a voice, the pitch of a stifled kiss, the feeling of a bright, open burst of laughter. Love is the simplicity of a person's ways, the essence and gracefulness of a being who, as this dream currently stands, answers to the name of Thomas. This same being kisses with his bright red lips and makes love with his loins arched. Leo caresses Thomas's neck with his fingers, which stray to his ears and the beginning of his hair. He closes his eyes and a peaceful smile spreads around his mouth. They are still sitting on the carpet, their backs against the wall, their legs outstretched. Leo is leaning over Thomas, kissing him and caressing every part of his face with his lips. Their embrace becomes tighter and closer as they yearn for total contact with each other. Their sexes touch like swords in a duel that is still tentative and ill-defined, blurred by their clothes. How long had it been since Leo had felt such a powerful, urgent desire as this? The smell of a young man, his hair, the light sweat on his back, the movements of a body surrendered to his strong arms, the quiver of muscles reacting to his powerful hands? Thomas is offering him all this with an inner readiness that Leo finds vibrant and mature.

He kneels beside Thomas's prostrate body. He gazes down at him, his eyes running up from his knees to his tapering thighs still hugged by his jeans. He stoops over his legs, stroking and kissing them. Then his eyes stray to Thomas's feet. He starts unlacing his shoes, first one then the other. He pulls off his socks and kisses his toes with his lips. He caresses Thomas's large, sculpted feet. He feels how soft the skin is, how dry and clean the toes, how taut his ankles. With his tongue he kisses the instep of each foot, holding them slightly raised off the floor in the cupped hollow of his hand. He strokes his own face with Thomas's feet, squeezing them hard.

Thomas stretches out his arms but cannot reach Leo crouched at his feet. His eyes open wider as desire wells up in him.

'Leo,' he murmurs, 'komme hier, mein Lieber komme.' Leo slowly looks up. His eyes meet Thomas's, staring wide, almost scared and timorous. 'I love you,' he says, his body arched above him.

'I love you,' Thomas repeats before he lets out a great sigh of abandonment and takes Leo's lips in his.

They stay like that for several minutes, rolling on the carpet towards the middle of the room. Leo feels Thomas's fingers trying to find his bare skin, unbuttoning his shirt and pulling it open. Then Leo gets up, puts one arm round Thomas's back and with the other grasps his legs. He flexes, braces himself and lifts Thomas bodily off the ground. Leo's heart beats faster, right where Thomas has rested his head. He moves towards the bed, just a few feet away in fact, although it feels like an eternity. He feels like a mother with a babe in arms. He feels Thomas arch his body as he holds on to his neck, trying to relieve him of some of the weight. He feels the tension in his own muscles, making him almost grit his teeth, but he wants to feel Thomas's weight, and the pleasure from Thomas's teeth and lips on his chest. Once by the bed he moves faster. Thomas laughs as he gets ready to be plunged down on to it. They fall hard on to the thick eiderdown, denting it as if they had landed in wet clay.

They lie close together again, entwined in the warmth of the bed. Maybe this first time together should stop right here. Something slackens momentarily in Leo's gaze, in the tension of his body. It could be no more than coyness, fear of what will happen next. Maybe it would be better to drop off to sleep just like this, breathing close together, keeping each other warm in Thomas's bed. But Leo knows he must make an effort, have his wits about him, and cope with the obstacle their love is putting in their way. Their attraction is definitely physical. It has to do with the beauty of their bodies, seductive glances, the flesh-pink colour of a cheek, or the suppleness of a move-ment. But it is something more, as well. A lot more. Now, in their total intimacy, this is why Leo is fearful about what is about to happen. He is afraid of spoiling every-thing, if they do not manage to find each other in the hardest test that is the collision between two bodies. It is the calm before the storm. But as if Thomas had sensed Leo holding himself back, he nestles close to him, fitting his body snugly beside Leo's. Thomas takes Leo's arms and wraps them round his chest, as if he were now carry-ing Leo on his back. Leo starts to thrust. Thomas guides him with the movements of his hips and with his hand.

Suddenly Leo realises he has come. He feels a slight ache in his groin, and a tight sensation that spreads up into his brain. A warm feeling. A comforting feeling of warmth and intimacy. He wants to say something, to find words for what he is feeling, to thank Thomas for what he has given him. But words dissolve in his mind. He knows they are there. He knows they play a crucial part in what is happening, but it is as if they cannot reach his lips. They are being pushed around the arena of his mind, faster and faster like lottery tickets in a drum. They drift hither and thither, bouncing and darting back and forth, but they cannot get out. And Leo realises that none of this makes any sense. The sense is in Thomas's body, in the panting hush that he is offering him, in the pleasure of finally being welcomed into another person's world.

The glimmer of first light filters into the room. Thomas is sleeping fitfully, fidgeting imperceptibly. His eyes open to find Leo standing silently by the bed, not sure what to do.

'Morning, Thomas,' Leo says quietly, his voice tremulous.

Thomas does not return the greeting. He turns his head slowly towards the arm where the hypodermic needle has been inserted. With what looks like a huge effort he checks the level of the glucose which is sustaining him. Leo draws near and touches Thomas's hand.

'How are you feeling?'

Thomas focuses his dark eyes on him. He pulls back the sheet and nods towards his stomach. A strip of white gauze and sticking plaster covers his body, from his groin to the centre of his chest. Some dark tubes emerge from the left side of his torso and disappear into the bed.

30

Thomas's father, standing at one corner of the bed, covers him up again with an instinctively prudish gesture of discretion. It was Thomas's father who phoned Leo to tell him in between sobs to come to Munich. 'My son wants to see you. Be quick. We don't have much time.'

Leo was at home in Milan. He drove all night straight to the clinic. The operation had taken place five days earlier, and it was five days before that that Thomas started having terrible pains in his stomach. Stabs of pain that seemed to flay his flesh. Heartburn that gnawed at his gut, like poison. And his whole abdomen was oddly, unnaturally swollen.

Leo never suspected he would find Thomas so worn out. He was obscenely thin, almost shrivelled. His face was sunken, the skin drawn tight over his cheekbones. His lips had almost vanished, reduced to a thin strip of skin barely covering his teeth. Head shaven. Arms and legs like an undernourished child's. And that huge belly, cut through and turned inside out. All that remains of the Thomas he has known is the eyes, if anything larger, wider and darker than ever. His eyes move wearily, almost motionless, the pupils just barely discernible. They are like two dark gaping holes, and they seem to repeat the same single thing, over and over: 'I can't, I can't believe this is happening to me.'

'Daddy, please let us be alone,' Thomas says. His voice is unrecognisable, a scarcely audible murmur. Faint and childlike, like a girl.

His father shakes his head, as if to ask why.

'I've got secrets,' Thomas says, smiling and trying to dilute his father's embarrassment. He uses a familiar password, probably referring to when he was a boy and he and his friends would steal away out of the reach of their parents 'for secret reasons'.

Thomas's father looks at his son, agreeing to leave the room. 'Only for five minutes, mind,' he adds.

They wait in silence as the man leaves. Once alone, Leo sits on the bed and lifts Thomas's hand to his face.

'Squeeze my hand, please,' Leo says. 'Squeeze it hard.'

'I've been so afraid of dying,' Thomas whispers staring out in front of him.

Leo swallows. He feels how hot Thomas's skin is. And he feels how far away Thomas is, too. It is as if the enormity of what he has had to go through has already killed him. As if terror had completely numbed him – that terror that is relentlessly invading him hour after hour. Leo has seen that same look on other occasions. The look of a Palestinian child about to be killed. The look of a little African baby dying beside its mother's body, mangled by bombs. The imploring gaze of a small Amazonian Indian child watching his race being wiped out. The look of people dying and begging hopelessly for help that will not come. Children, children. And Thomas the child, turning again to his father, like he did all those years ago. 'I'll see you're soon out of here. The worst is over. Try and get some strength back. I'll take you to Spain. We'll stay in the Grand Hotel in Saragossa and play bingo. Anything you like . . . *Comencemos, primero número el sesenta y nueve, seis y nueve. Luego el ochenta y siete, ocho y siete. ¡Línea! . . . ¡Han cantado línea!*'. For years they made each other laugh by repeating these words, and spelling out all the bingo numbers.

Now Leo attempts a smile, but with little heart.

'Are you really doing okay?' Thomas breaks in.

Leo is embarrassed by his own fit body. He is tempted to say no, no I'm not doing okay at all, my love. But he knows he must put on a brave face. He knows that Thomas is aware of what is going on. Then he feels a need to touch him in a different way. He uncovers his legs and gently strokes them, working up from the knee to his bare buttocks. He fondles his sex and his shaven groin. 'You're still as sexy as ever, Thomas,' he says finally.

Thomas turns his head away and his eyelids lower slowly.

Leo pulls the sheet back over him.

Thomas's father comes back in. Leo realises he should leave. In this last moment, Thomas is back in the family fold, with the very same people who brought him into the world. Now, with their hearts torn asunder by suffering, they are trying to help Thomas to die. There is no room for Leo in this parental reconciliation. Leo is not married to Thomas. He has not had children with him. Neither of them bears the other's name at the registry office, and there is not a single legal record on the face of the earth that carries the signatures of witnesses to their union. Yet for more than three years they have been passionately in love with one another. They have lived together in Paris and Milan, and they have travelled round Europe together. They have written together, played music together and danced together. They have quarrelled and abused each other, and even hated each other. They have been in love. But it is as if, without warning, beside that deathbed, Leo realised that he had experienced not a great love story, but rather some little school crush. As if they were telling him: You've both had a good time, and that's okay too. But here we're fighting a life and death struggle. Here a life is at stake. And we – a father, a mother and a son – are what really matters in life.

Then Leo feels everything about his own life separated by a yawning chasm from the great moments of life and death. As if he has always lived in some other part of society. As if his unhappiness or happiness in the world, his wanderings, everything had taken place on a stage. Now the performance had come to an end. Fathers and mothers, the church, the state, the registrar of deaths, all were laying claim to what was theirs. They were putting things back in order, burying and committing everything to the dust of archives, the dust that reduces it all to nought. All of it except the insignificant grief of a young stranger.

Leo presses Thomas's father's hand. He looks him straight in the eye. His face is Thomas's face. If Thomas had lived to be fifty he would perhaps have looked like this, a tall, handsome man with an air of distinction about him, a slight stoop of the shoulder, and those incredible eyebrows, bushy and black. But Thomas is dying. He is twenty-five. And Leo, who is only four years older, Leo is about to become the widower of a partner like no other. And there are no words to express it. There is no human utterance that can define the person who, for him, has been not a husband, not a wife, not a lover, not just a companion, but the crucial part of a new, shared destiny.

He looks back at Thomas at the far end of the room and says goodbye. He says: 'See you soon. Get better soon.' But Thomas does not answer. He does not say a word to him. He looks at him with his huge, enormous dark eyes, clinging desperately, with dread and terror, to the figure who is about to walk out of his life forever. Leo cannot stand the sight of those gaping eyes a moment more. They are all he can see. The whole room is Thomas's eyes. He lowers his head and leaves, still muttering the odd word to suit the occasion. He knows full well that he will carry within him, for as long as he lives, that look from Thomas the manchild on his deathbed in his separate room.

He returns to Milan once more by night. His car floats along the almost deserted roads until he is back home. He lets himself in, turns on the light, and goes to the kitchen. He sits down with a glass of beer. He smokes a cigarette, then a second and a third and a fourth, staring at the black television screen. The things around him seem new, that at least is how they appear to his unusually heavy eyes. He realises, almost for the very first time, that there is a pair of valuable Chinese vases on the dresser. A film of dust shrouds the tins of Indian tea. The rubber plant, more than six feet tall, needs watering. Maybe he should spray its leaves.

Beyond the small terrace the dark wall of the huge building opposite shuts out the sky. The vast wall of windows is unlit and dark. A solemn silence hangs there. Among the hundreds and hundreds of people sleeping just a few yards away, Leo is the only one who knows that Thomas is dying. Even if he does not want it to change, not for anything in the world, his life is changing. And he has no idea whatsoever what direction it might go in. He feels as if he should do a shift of sentry duty. He is tired, has no energy. Ahead lies a dark, lonely night, gripping a rifle and waiting for the enemy who will not come, waiting for thieves or terrorists who will never appear under his watch-tower. There is no desire in him for anything. He is alone, in the darkness, with his own dread. The eyes which saw death just a few hours ago, these same eyes no longer see things the same way.

Years and years ago, when he was not much more than twenty, something similar had perhaps happened. And as he grew older, he had realised that that particular event had been nothing other than the traumatic and extremely violent conquest of the barrier keeping him locked up in his adolescence, in his myths and in his illusions. He had realised almost overnight that he was suddenly a man. He was no longer a boy, and he was no longer immortal. The person who had always seen death as a friend to talk to on dark school days – when no one else seemed interested in taking him tenderly in their arms, this same person was suddenly terrified of dying. He saw himself dead, and conscious of it. It was more than he could bear.

He was driving fast in an old Opel along the straight, narrow country lanes that criss-cross the wide countryside of the Po Valley like a huge spider's web. With him in the car were two young men about whom he knew absolutely nothing. The aroma of grapes just harvested still hung on the air, and the mist rising through the autumn sunset from irrigation ditches and ponds looked like the slow breathing of the earth about to fall asleep. The leaves of the poplars and elms lining the roadside were turning yellow. He had leaned out of the window, defying the cold. The others were singing along with the rock music on the radio. The driver was as thin as a pole, with long dirty hair, and wearing jeans. He was wearing a pair of small glasses held together in more places than one by strips of tape that were now grimy black, and sticky. He had a wispy beard on the tip of his chin and sideburns. Some of his teeth were missing, creating a dark window in his mouth. When he spoke, the words came out garbled in a way that amused Leo. Despite this, he had already managed to open three small bottles of beer with his molars, spitting the metal caps out of the window, along with a little blood mingling with the white froth of the beer.

The other passenger was good-looking and well-built, with a crew-cut. He was doing his military service, and he was on convalescent leave. He had picked up lice or scabies or something like that. He had reddish scabs on his wrists and legs. He had to use a foul-smelling cream. But he did not seem too bothered by it all.

Leo had met them in the bar behind the old theatre, in town. He was drinking some kind of liquor. He had hair down to his shoulders, and not a penny to his name. A local girl, just out of jail, had sidled up to him and asked where she could score some drugs, fast. Leo replied with a shrug of the shoulders but the girl would not let up. Then when the toothless wonder and the louse-infected conscript turned up, everything happened in just a matter of minutes. They all leapt into the car and sped off. Leo had the girl's 50,000 lire in his pocket. She did not want to trust the other two with her money. They, for their part, with their clean records, did not want to get involved with the girl because she had a police record.

They headed off to make a small deal. Low quality dope was doing the rounds of the bars, helping people to make a little money so they could pay for better stuff when the hard stuff came through. Nothing had been coming through for months, and now there was this shipment forty miles away, in some isolated place by the Po. Why Leo had agreed without a second thought to go along in the car, he could not rightly say: he did not use drugs, at least not hard drugs.

His imagination had been stirred and that was reason enough.

He might have wanted to write about it: go along for the ride, see the deal for himself, and then come back and tell what he had seen. He was twenty and he needed stories. But the real reason why he went along would blow up dangerously in his face, just a few hours later. It was nothing more than a car ride, for a couple of hours, on an excruciating autumn day with the sun still high in the sky. There was beer and music, and something to see. The only danger was the police, but he knew how to look after himself, and he would never let himself be found with anything on him – he would not even touch the stuff. An hour to get there, an hour to do the deal, and another hour to get back. An exciting little adventure and no reason why not. Everything was in order.

The car was speeding along the deserted country roads and he was breathing in the sacred air of his native land. He felt on top of the world, and he felt right. He would never have imagined that, as it turned out, it would take him years and years to make the trip back.

They reached their destination with the sun already hidden behind a line of poplars. They parked the car down a track. At the end of it stood a farmhouse. There were no cars, no lights, just silence, and now it was dark.

'Are you sure this is the place?' Leo asked, disappointed.

The driver did not answer.

'Shit! You sure this is the place?' the other one yelled from behind. He got out of the car and slammed the door. He pulled out his cock and pissed in the road.

'This is the place, sure,' the toothless wonder stammered.

'They must have changed places. Maybe something's gone wrong, who knows?'

The other man got back into the car cursing and swearing.

Leo started to feel uneasy. He realised that this little trio of perfect strangers could break up from one moment to the next. He said something like let's wait a bit, somebody's bound to show up, but he did not say it with much conviction. The toothless wonder opened the last remaining bottle of beer his way. He nicked his lip and spat blood. A few moments later a car pulled up with its headlights dimmed. Two men got out. They approached cautiously. Before anyone spoke they took a good look at Leo's face and the faces of the other two, who had wound down the windows and were sitting there motionless. Like animals sniffing each other up and down, they were not sure whether to trust each other or not. Then one of them said: 'I know you, you're a friend of Riccio's, aren't you?'

The one with the teeth missing nodded. 'Shit, there's nobody here,' he said after a while.

'Maybe they're at Bachi's then,' said the other. 'It's not far.'

'Who's Bachi?' said the man sitting behind Leo.

No one answered. 'Let's try going over there,' he went on, leaning on the window. 'You guys coming?'

The one with the teeth missing started the car.

Bachi's place was not exactly a house. It was a restored railway inspector's lodge. It stood in the middle of a wide expanse of countryside where there were no trees. From the road all you could see was the small building, far off, but no access road leading to it. The disused railway tracks ran alongside the tarmac road. There was practically no ballast. It seemed to be more like a narrow-gauge track. It was slightly higher than the level of the road, with grass growing between the rails. They eventually found an unmade-up track to turn down. It was not much more than three feet wide. The car wheels had to fit into two deep ruts left by heavy farm machinery. A hundred yards further on, they found a metal bar and a rusty sign that said 'Keep Out'. Leo felt a sense of foreboding, but it only lasted a split second. They left the car behind a small building out of sight of the road. There were two other cars there and a motorbike. A window opened and a voice hailed them through the dark, telling them to come on in. Leo said he would wait in the car. He reckoned the others would be back in a few minutes, without getting what they had gone in for. But half an hour went by. Then an hour. The silence was unreal and disconcerting. Nobody came out of the house. There was not a sound. No lights, nothing. Leo got out of the car and banged on the door. Nothing. He started to get worried. The cars were still there . . . But why so long? And why didn't anyone come and tell him what was going on? He knocked louder. The upstairs window opened and a dim light lit up the half-rubbed out words 'Signal Box No. 84'.

'What's going on?' Leo shouted at the stranger. 'What's happened to those two guys?'

The window closed again and someone came down-stairs to open the door. Leo decided he would go upstairs. He found himself in a large room with a few mattresses on the floor, Indian fabrics hanging on the walls, and dirty cushions, torn and stained, scattered here and there. There were two mangy old dogs shuffling about among the people sprawled on the floor. There were cups full of ash and cigarette butts, incense burning, open boxes of medicine, and a pot of tea doing the rounds. There were about ten people in all. Leo realised that at least half of them were stoned out of their minds. There was a strong smell of hashish. A few people were smoking. But there was too much tinfoil being passed around not to realise that these people had been putting something else into their veins.

Leo went over to the guy with the car and said it was time to go. He nodded and then looked blank again. Leo shivered and his legs started to shake. He felt uncomfort-able. Worse, he felt sick. He took a couple of puffs and swigged at some greenish concoction. He felt a pleasant warm sensation in his stomach and took another swig. He started to relax. All the tension he had built up in the car, and earlier when they went to the wrong house, started to fade. He felt good, took another puff at the pipe, then chewed on some brown leaves. He took another swig of the green stuff and smoked some more. The faces all around him seemed a bit more friendly now and a bit more familiar, too. He felt himself letting go. After all, he could stay all night feeling like this. He saw himself chatting with the others until morning. He was on the point of letting his imagination take over when a sudden thought struck him. It was a strange sensation, and one that was merely irksome to begin with. But later it became harder to put up with. It was a malaise that grew within him and it felt as heavy as a block of meat. He tried to remember, but could not. The faces around him started to turn less friendly, becoming harder and more and more unpleasant. They were corrupting him. The lotus eaters were diverting him from his mission. Then he remembered: he had to get back home to take the stuff back to that girl. He could not spend the night in this place, with all these stinking mattresses smelling of dog's piss and people slumped all over the floor, people who wanted to kill him. He had to get back home, so he could write. He had a task to complete. These were not his kind of people, he had to get back to his kind of people as soon as possible. That is how he started to feel cold, colder and colder. Like a shudder that shook him harder and harder to the very marrow in his bones. He started to shiver all over. He looked about him, but nobody seemed to realise what was happening to him. He went to the good-looking man who smelt of insecticide and said to him: 'Did you get the stuff?'

'What stuff?'

'The shit, for Christ's sake!' Leo screamed.

The one who must have been Bachi, an almost bald man of about thirty with a long beard, said: 'Something the matter, kid? This is my house. So why not tell me if something's the matter?'

Leo drew closer to him. 'I came in the car with these two guys. I've got to get back. I can't stay here. Did you give them the stuff? Okay, so let's go. This isn't the way we agreed to do it. We've been driving around all afternoon.'

Bachi looked at him and touched his arm. 'What stuff?'

Leo closed his eyes and felt he was going crazy. He tried to stay calm. 'You haven't got anything here?' he said, almost begging.

'The stuff's coming in first thing at dawn. We're all waiting. Stay cool. In a while we'll go and clinch the deal.'

'I can't wait!' Leo shouted. He paced around the room. His ideas felt more and more confused and remote. He could not think straight any more. He did not understand what he was doing with all these people, but he still managed to remember that he had to get back home. There was something that he had to do, but before long he forgot what. It was just at that moment, when he lost track of himself, that the trip began. He trembled all over, he was sweating, and felt a need to run. He dashed outside and started to run wildly round and round the building, faster and faster. The moon was high in the sky. Bright as bright, and huge. Leo could see his own shadow. He felt frightened and tried to hide. But he could not. He ran along the track and reached the tarmac road. He ran on and on. The poplars flashed by fast on either side of him. He felt like he was running at a hundred miles an hour. Then he realised he was running harder and harder, stronger and stronger, and there was no speed that could compare with the speed of his thoughts which kept coming and coming and then dying, one after the other, and he did not understand, he kept asking and asking, always asking questions in his attempt to understand, but now millions of other problems and faces and ideas and situations were bursting in his brain and there was nothing that could stop them. He prayed and begged, as he ran on and on, that he could stop, stop for a split second at just one idea or just one thought, but it was not possible. The dizziness of it all dragged him into a whirlpool where there was no top or bottom, no above or below, dragged him inside the very idea of vertigo, into the very essence of a word which did not exist. When he finally saw this – because he no longer managed to grasp or understand or realise anything, all he could do was see with his eyes covered – he experienced a moment of horror. He raised his eyes towards the night and he was all of a sudden in orbit. Everything exploded all about him. He was inside a missile being fired into space, travelling faster and faster, burning up millions of billions of light years, and he was inside it, running, and running, and running faster and faster. He saw the earth far away, reduced to a tiny blackish dot swallowed up by the darkness of the night, but what earth was he seeing? He was not of this world. He felt he never had been of this world. He had no parents, no children. He had no one who loved him, no one who could hold him down on earth, no one who was coming with him on this journey. He was alone, lost at interstellar speed, in the darkness of the firmament, being propelled further and further away, to ever greater distances. Forever.

He ran on even faster, leaving the road and taking to the fields. He did not feel tired. He could not feel the beating of his own heart. He did not feel his own breath chilling his teeth. He felt neither cold nor hot, well nor ill. He was too immeasurably far away. He stumbled into a ditch. There was not much water in it, six inches or so of muddy sludge, already freezing over. He started to walk, following the ditch. He was moving slowly now, and his thoughts had slowed down too. He had no idea how much time had passed. But passed since when? When had this whole story started? And what kind of story was it? His story? Or the Other's story? But who was he? He was himself through and through, but at the same time he was nobody. Nobody. He felt himself going out of his mind, once, ten times, and a hundred million times. In his brain he could feel the cells burning up. He could feel them glowing red hot and endlessly sprouting one into the other, sizzling and spurting, dying and dissolving, and always a million more nerve ends coming on. He could feel the hum and buzz of neurons darting madly hither and thither in a labyrinth that had no sides. A labyrinth that was confined within his finite body, but that even so would never have any limits. Smaller and smaller, deeper and deeper, until he reached the universe, and those astral limits that he felt coming closer and closer, nearer and nearer. And then, when he had reached the place beyond – and now he could see the light, because way beyond the limits there was a light – he would fling himself over and never, never come back.

He started to cry. He fell down and cried. The light was coming closer and he did not want to fall into it. He wanted to brake, to stop where he was. He did not want to reach the edge of the universe. He wanted to die and find peace. But he was already dead and he knew that there was no peace there, either. The light was growing brighter and brighter, whiter and whiter, until he yelled even louder and felt a roar and an unbearable pain in his temples. 'No! No!' he screamed, but the words were like explosions, one after the other. Everything was exploding and the light was more and more blinding. The blackness of the sky had vanished.

Suddenly he could see himself, from the outside maybe, and from a long way off, but he could still see himself. He saw himself in that ditch and it was as if he recognised himself again. He tried to hold on to what he was feeling, to what he was touching with his hands. He tried to cling to what he was bringing up to his mouth. It had a marshy, muddy, swampy smell about it, but it was a smell he could remember and place in a 'real' vision. He drank that water and called it water, and he called the mud mud and started to feel a little better. He had cut himself and he touched what he could have sworn was called blood, and for him it could be clearly related to that word, but there was no 'blood'. There was something else that people had called blood but that he, at that moment in time, knew with absolute, razor-edge certainty to have always had another name.

Things were becoming enormous inside of him. They

were pulling the nails out of his senses and making them jump. His own senses and the sense of reality and the sense of that unreality that words are. Like all people, all he had to keep him on earth was words. Their therapy would put him right. He begged them not to leave him.

He came to the high street of a small town. There was no one around. He walked close up against the walls, colliding every so often with the pillars of the colonnades. He found himself looking at a public noticeboard about five feet long. It was made of iron, rusting at one corner, and it held the opened pages of a newspaper. A small mesh metal grid held the pages in place. He started to read, understanding not a word. He read out loud, starting from the very first word and spelling everything out, commas, full stops, paragraphs, capital letters, the lot, trying to create a small pool of light for himself with the soaked matches in his pocket, and using his fingertips, scratched by the metal mesh, to keep his place. He stayed several hours there. The fog had reached the town and wafted beneath the arcades as if blown in by a turbine. He knew it was time to go.

He left the town, taking more country roads until he felt a sense of huge, enormous suspension, between the earth and the sky and the river. Day was dawning, the stars were small translucent dots, twinkling prettily. He took a deep breath and saw that he had reached the mouth of the river.

He undressed on the cold, dirty beach. He gathered twigs and driftwood and old newspapers and lit a small fire. He walked towards the water, completely naked, washed and went back to the fire. Everything he did, every gesture and every action, was somehow automatic. He could make no decisions about anything. But he could see himself doing things, and this activity made him feel better. Everything was born from the sea. And now he had returned to the sea. The glimmer in the sky grew brighter. He looked at the water and saw millions of beings being born there and being washed up on to the beach by the waves, and then vanishing when a million more beings were about to be washed up in turn. He was one of those beings. He was a small transparent cell with a nucleus pulsating away inside. With the next wave he became a molecule, and with the one after a complete entity. Then he was an animal, then another animal – but he was still himself, he was quite sure of that. Until everything fell quiet and nothing and no one came up out of the sea any more.

He thought of his mother and wept. He thought of his mother's mother, and the mother of his mother's mother. He felt marooned. He wept some more. He saw himself like an aborted foetus, tossed from one womb to another over millions of years. There was no longer any No one, no longer any Nothingness. There was an individual being that suffered as it grew. Then he thought that all these images of mothers, and of mothers' laps, and then images of languages that he had learnt, were nothing other than the figures of an incarnation. He thought he was going back home, and this gave him confidence. He was becoming himself again, there on the seashore, in his own story. He was descending down into himself and this wordless, mute descent was happening like an endless adjustment of perspective. At one and the same time he was millions

48

of lives, but always, and more so, just one life. He did not want to understand anything any more. He was terrified at the thought of trying to stop these visions he had been having hours, or centuries, or even whole epochs ago. He gave in to whatever was coming out of his head. It was distress. But a different kind of distress to the dread that had almost done him in just a few hours earlier. What had happened was that, in his own biological substance, he had experienced cosmic solitude. He had experienced confusion and Nothingness. And he had asked this Nothingness for an explanation, thinking like a pebble, a river, a tree or a fish. But now his distress was the same distress that is in billions of other people. In a certain sense it was embodied in a kind of universe. He was no longer in a state of absolute delirium of being, living or existing. Rather he was in a delirium of knowing, from the moment when he had touched base on the seashore, that he was definitely not dead – contrary to what he had believed a few hours, or centuries, or even whole epochs ago. And his journey down to earth passed through images of women and women's laps and languages.

Layer upon layer of words came and covered him over, protecting him and keeping him warm. The schoolmistress was leaning over him, holding him by the arm and helping him gently with a gesture that miraculously wrote down on the sheet of paper, with ink, an idea, a sensation, a world. And he could smell the scent of his schoolmistress's lipstick and it entranced him. The words which formed in front of his boy's eyes held the perfume of the teacher's lips, as soon as they had been scribbled on the paper with the pen. His mother came to fetch him from school. She was on her bicycle. She was wearing a white apron and a small bag of warm bread was hanging from the handlebars. He ran towards her. She took the piece of paper and put him in his seat. She asked him how things had gone on his first day at school and he laughed as he looked at her. He saw her lips and he wanted to kiss her. He felt a sweet, sweet feeling of delight because it seemed to him that those first words he had written had a flavour of bread and the scent of nice lipstick about them.

He stayed there beside the sea, not moving, for hours and hours, immune to the cold, to hunger and to tiredness. He could not feel his body and his movements became increasingly tiring and lazy, and slower and slower. Later, with no clue how he came to be where he was – he remembered an electric train swaying through the countryside and a man driving a truck – he knew for sure that he was on the way home, that he was getting nearer and nearer to a place where he could rest and be at peace. And it was a smell that led him back home. A smell that made him realise that he was getting there, that the journey, or at least that extreme part of his journey, was about to end. The smell was strong as it came through the mist fragrant with wine and dank land. He puffed out his lungs and walked bent over so that he could better hold on to the smell. It was the smell of his country, a land where there were more pigs than people. It was a smell of pigsties and sows and their dung collected in huge tanks to be converted into energy. Sows. More pigs than people. There, on the banks of the mouth of the river Po, Leo knew that his childhood was over, and he was painfully aware that he was just one of the millions of beings this was happening to. He was no longer a boy. He had tried to ask questions and understand, and, tormented by this need to know, he had pushed his luck too far. He had travelled to the very edge of the abyss and turned back in total disarray. Now he no longer knew anything for certain. He had no answers. But from now on he would ask no more questions either. He would have to remake himself, day by day. He would have to re-learn, in a different way, everything he used to know, because absurdity had erased all trace of the past in him. In some way he was a brand new person. Or maybe one Leo had simply died and a different one had been born. He would no longer study philosophy, or eastern religions, or Hebrew, or the mystics of the Middle Ages. He would no longer ask questions about the ultimate meaning of things, because he had proved that no such meaning existed, and that if ever a final meaning might appear, from somewhere or other, it would just be chaos, and people would just be players in a small, senseless game, whose numerical savagery nobody would ever be able to comprehend. But for all that it was just a game, and all games are based on rules which make them possible. Leo would learn the rules. He would obey them and accept them. He would never dig his heels in again. He had done away with the absolute.

So it was that the new Leo grew, and grew stronger, day by day and year by year. The way he looked at things had changed radically. He was the same person, but he carried within him the bloody marks of an abortion, of a Leo who had been burnt. Deep within him he retained the

51

scars and breaks of the other Leo. And every so often, as he followed the rules like an obedient little schoolboy, he reopened the scars and breaks, and moved them about. And only by this shifting from place to place did he manage to find a bit of peace.

On this other night, fraught with thoughts of Thomas dying, Leo feels that everything is changing yet again. He seemed to have reached a state of equilibrium with his friend, but now all the cards are on the table once more. And in the cruellest way. In a few days he will once again be even more alone on his path through life. And this time he does not know how the deep and sacred mourning that he is carrying within him for the first time might change him. He will have to start his night watch. With tears in his eyes he takes his head in his hands and utters the syllables of Thomas's name, as if to hold him still close to him. Hundreds of miles apart, one of them confined to his hospital bed, and the other sitting as if petrified on a hard chair in his kitchen, they are both young men with an unspeakable fear of dying.

SECOND MOVEMENT

Leo's World

Each year autumn ushers in the same feelings. A need for silence and solitude and recollection. A need to sleep. To take stock. A need for introspection. The earth summons him unto her and invites him to gather his thoughts. And Leo, born in the glow of a late summer's day, covered deep down with dark soil, odours of rotting leaves, and swamps, and mists, Leo hears this summons and follows it. One morning towards the end of summer he sets off from home on a journey.

He gives vague answers when friends ask why he is going off, and tries to make them seem believable. He says he is going away to work. He will be going to London to write a few articles, and he will be back in a few months. He is forced to lie to parry the slightly worried concern of people who are fond of him. He feels imprisoned by the common sense of his friends, who would never go off travelling without organising their journey and reserving in advance. He sees how concerned they are. He senses how awkward they feel as they carefully avoid asking him the one question they would really like to ask him: 'What's happening to you, Leo? It's serious, isn't it?' And he goes on lying and hedging, straying from the point and giving them addresses he will never be at, just to keep them quiet.

In fact he is lying because he knows full well how fragile his own reasons really are. All he knows is that he must get on the road. He does not know what to do with himself any more. He would like to sleep for years, a thousand years, laid out in a hushed wood, on a bed of bright yellow leaves, or red leaves like the vines in October, or orange leaves like Canadian maples, or violet like flesh. And wake up again quite different. He would like to walk in silence across mountains, with just the rustle of his own footsteps and his own breathing. He would like to feel within him the smell of the soil stirring at dawn, soil forever breaking up and rotting. He would like to vanish, sucked up by the vapours of a fuming bog. He would like never to return from his journey. He would like to get lost on a dead-end track and disappear without trace.

He does not have any precise destination. He plans to travel at a leisurely pace, by train, across Europe. He will avoid major towns and capital cities. He will stay overnight in small provincial towns, and spend time sitting at tables in local taverns and pubs and bars. He will turn in early to sleep, and wake up every day before it gets light. He has bought a railpass that is valid for three months. He has packed everything he will need into three bags. He is taking just one book with him. He intends to read it line by line, like the verses of the Bible. He has a notebook for jotting things down and a Walkman for listening to music. This way he feels better equipped for his expedition beyond the confines of Thomas's body.

Across the continent autumn is putting on a dazzling display. There is stillness and silence. The forests are bursting with colours and the dying undergrowth ignites a whole range of hues, first red, then orange, yellow, russet, violet and black. As if each day the wind pushed a different shade into the air, and bushes and plants absorbed that coloured air in waves. And every so often there were whole hillsides scorched by acid rain. Trees already like skeletons, black and emaciated and charred. Now he is making his way across the Rhineland. The river is full and metallic grey. The barges chug slowly along, looking to Leo as if they are about to sink. He shuts his eyes. With Thomas, once, he had driven by car along the very road now running parallel with the train. It was spring. April, perhaps. And they were heading for Cologne. Leo had gone to see Thomas in Munich, where his family lived. They had slept together at the Deutsche Eiche.

They drank many beers in the tavern, sitting on wooden benches, close to a huge old stove covered with majolica tiles, beneath a ceiling filled with coloured balloons. They were surrounded by dozens of men aged between thirty and fifty, wearing black leather trousers and short leather waistcoats decorated with studs and chains, and black t-shirts pulled tight across their bulging bellies. Their beards were dripping with beer. There was laughter. A lot of them were wearing cheap earrings and junk jewellery. Some were wearing short Tyrolean lederhosen, too. The older men among them gently rocked their paunches, arms locked with the people sitting beside them. The younger men ordered drinks, calling for the waiter who wore a pair of net stockings, very high heels, a black moustache, and a leather waistcoat. People slapped him on the butt, and the waiter tried to dodge them, moving like a belly-dancer. He laughed a lot, shouted a few quips, and carried on with his show sitting on the knees of the 'leather men'.

What was happening at the Deutsche Eiche that night, as had happened on thousands of other nights, was the ritual of a community. The postures and attitudes, the gestures and words, the clothes, the boots and the studs, all of it was part and parcel of a ceremonial rite. Leo felt profoundly removed from it, but at the same time he felt as if he belonged there. And if he kept a close eye on the way people behaved, and if he basically felt at ease in that place, it was because he was aware of the way a minority group deals with the problem of its own differences. And even if he felt alien to the ceremonies, and to what might well seem almost like a melancholy perversion when seen from the outside, he simply appreciated the fact that it existed. He did not take part in the performance. But he acknowledged the reasons for it. And in acknowledging it he could justify it.

He kept up with Thomas passing the tankard round after round, once, twice, five times, until he finally started to feel drunk. He watched his friend singing or chatting with other people. They went on drinking, and started to add Steinhäger to the beer. Then they went into the

56

kitchen, asked for the room number, and walked up to the second floor. There were no keys. And on the way Leo saw several rooms with the door open and people on the bed, in the red glow from the lampshade, making love or beckoning to him to come along in. The rooms had no telephone or heating or cupboards. The bathroom was a tiny, icy cubicle, and the peephole of a window, giving on to a courtyard, had broken panes of glass and a peeling frame. They took off their clothes and hurriedly got under the duvet. They were freezing cold. They kissed and hugged each other.

The next day someone had knocked insistently at the door.

A man walked in and gave them a friendly wake-up call. They left Munich around eleven that morning. Thomas was at the wheel of his dilapidated Citroën. He drove with one hand and held Leo's hand with the other. Every now and then he lifted Leo's hand to his lips. Leo was map-reading.

They reached Cologne. That evening, at dinner, Leo met one or two academics, a secretary at the Italian embassy, and a couple of German journalists. They talked about a literary festival. Leo used Thomas as his interpreter. And when they spoke in Italian it was Leo's turn to translate. He sensed how the other men all seemed to be permanently wondering what kind of relationship there was between him and Thomas. Leo sensed this from the way they looked at him in the lulls during the conversation, and from the way they behaved with slight embarrassment towards Thomas, because they were not sure of his role.

One day a friend had said to him: 'I never go on my own when they invite me. It's normal that if you invite a fifty-year-old fellow like me to a dinner, or a festival, or a meeting, he takes his wife along too. Well, I've had a partner for twenty-five years. And for twenty-five years he's been coming along with me to receptions and meetings. Vice versa, too: I go along with him when he's the one who's invited. It's the least we can do. We mustn't let them invite us on our own.'

Ever since Leo had heard these words for the first time he had lived up to them, as if they were some kind of revelation. Of course there was always the risk of misunderstanding. Not to mention embarrassment. When he explained that he would not be alone and the haughty voice came back from the other end of the telephone line: 'But of course, do bring your wife along too,' and when he then pointed out that he would be accompanied by Mister such-and-such and that the hotel room should be registered under his name as well, there would be a silence, a clearing of the throat, and a cough interrupting the conversation like a tangible gesture of embarrassment. He would then calmly explain that he had arranged to travel with his friend, but had not organised his hotel accommodation. Then the bureaucrat would hastily end their conversation with a meek 'As you wish.'

In Cologne, as in other cities where Leo had been accompanied by Thomas, curiosity about who this young man was would hang over the conversation. Neither Leo nor Thomas had effeminate ways. Neither of them fitted what was expected of a homosexual. They were not histrionic, they were not show-offs, they did not make a noise, they were not vulgar, and they were not forever talking about sex. They defied easy definition and this added to other people's embarrassment. The outcome of it all was that officials and academics, for whom all that matters is appearances and bureaucratic formalities, went on wondering, behind their polite smiles, whether these two young men were or were not.

The next leg of that journey took them to Duisberg, where Leo gave a short lecture at the university. Thomas sat at his side, his seat set slightly behind Leo's. He would lean forward, brushing against the nape of Leo's neck, to translate the students' questions into French. Leo listened to Thomas's lips giving him the gist of what was being said. Every so often he would turn round to ask Thomas to explain something again, and he would watch Thomas sitting there, bent forward, serious, intent on understanding the precise nature of a question, although the only reason for Thomas's interest in the question was because it was part of Leo's life. And in those moments Leo wondered if he would have been able to do the same for Thomas – get passionately involved in his life, stay close by him, suggest the boundaries of a problem, and help him to get along in the world with other people. And he did not know for sure. He felt a kind of imbalance between the devotion that Thomas was showing him and the devotion that he was capable of showing Thomas. Day in day out, his life had become Thomas's life. And maybe this is what Leo had wanted. But what did he really know about his partner? He knew he was the son of a modest Bavarian clerk. He knew he had two older brothers and a French Swiss mother who had once been a musician. He knew Thomas was studying at the Conservatoire in Paris. He knew he preferred making love some ways more than others. He knew how he stared at him hard and said with his serious, concentrated voice, 'I know those eyes of yours already, Leo.' He knew that before he had met him, Thomas was living with a girl. He knew he liked beer and tobacco. So many little details, some more telling than others. But Leo had still not entered fully into the life of this other person. Maybe because he had had other affairs and was more experienced. Maybe because he was more cautious and reluctant about letting a new destiny take him over. There were nights spent sleeping with Thomas when he would suddenly open his eyes and see Thomas staring stiffly out into space. He would move closer to him and ask him what he was thinking about, and Thomas would give a scared answer, as if he were about to panic: 'Who are you? Who am I sleeping with?' And Leo realised that in that moment Thomas was not really asking him who he was. He realised that Thomas was asking what kind of strange significance there was about him sharing his bed with a stranger. And because Leo had no answer to this question, Thomas could not bring himself to move, because he was frightened by a feeling of separation and loss, his eyes were wide-open and staring, and all he could do was wonder why he was lying next to a torturer, a persecutor who was cruelly robbing him of his own being.

Then Leo would force himself not to touch Thomas. He would get up, switch on the light, toss a few words at Thomas, open the window, and read a page from a book out loud in an attempt to bring Thomas back to the reality that had disappeared in fear between their two bodies. And when he saw that Thomas was past the critical moment, he would go over to him and simply squeeze his hand, with the words: 'We need time. We need to put in some time together. We need to live together, travel together, so that the way each of us thinks is instinctively tuned to the way the other is thinking. Like an automatic response of familiarity and affection. We need a lot of time to accept the brutal fact that we're not alone any more.'

But in Duisberg that night it was Leo's turn not to sleep.

They had been together just over six months. They had met in November, and now they were discovering their first spring together. For that whole brief period Leo had tried as best he could to respond to Thomas's needs. He had involved Thomas in his own life. He had cheered him up, and protected him. He had restrained him from going over the top, and encouraged him in moments of doubt. He thought that the success of their relationship had to do more or less exclusively with the way Thomas behaved. For his part, he felt a certain calm within him. He wanted Thomas for life itself. He was not looking for adventures. There was time. He would say to himself, let's give it a try for a few years, let's try to stay together because we want to. And just a few days after he had got to know Thomas, Thomas had said to him: 'I want to live with you forever, Leo.' So their quarrels and rows were always somehow delimited within a territory from which they knew they could not escape. They squabbled and fought. Sometimes they would not speak to each other for days. One of them would stomp off and the other would call up old friends. But it never lasted more than a few days. They always ended up getting back together again. And what played a crucial part in this was their sexual chemistry, and the mutual physical attraction between them. They were turned on by each other. They desired each other. And they needed to find one another again.

Throughout those months their relationship had been structured by Leo. Thomas invested his enthusiasm in it, but it was Leo who felt he was controlling it. And it was Leo, if anyone, who felt he could be done with it as and when he wished. But that night in Duisberg, it was Leo who felt trapped. Trapped by seeing himself absorbed by Thomas, who was still very young, and had no job, no career and no security. Thomas was just beginning to develop. He still had to decide what to do with his life. Leo had taken years and years to put together something resembling a normal existence. He had suffered and gone through the mill. And he had put up with it. And now here he was once more getting involved with something that was uncertain and risky. But he could not stop himself. He was too aware of Thomas's devotion to him. He felt it too deeply. This time around he had been touched in a spot that he had not thought Thomas could get to so fast. And everything had happened in that university lecture-hall seething with hundreds of students who had applauded him for what seemed like endless minutes, banging their fists on the wooden benches in their traditional way. He had felt stirred and moved by that wall of faces in front of him in the lecture-hall, all noisily showing their approval of what he had said, the points he had made, his answers to their questions, and the way a particular topic of discussion had fired him. Those students banging the benches in the hall were on his side.

Leo turned towards the long table lined with professors.

To his surprise he saw that they, too, were banging the table with their fists and giving him affable smiles of satisfaction. And even officialdom, in the form of the Italian consul with his blue ribbon and a huge ring on his little finger and his old-fashioned airs of a southern gentleman, was clapping his hands. Even the cultural attaché at the Italian embassy, who had come all the way from Bonn, was applauding him from the front row of the auditorium. And if there had been a general or a police commissioner, Leo was quite sure they would have joined in the applause as well. Even a judge, even the Law would have banged on the benches in approval. He turned and amid that hullabaloo saw Thomas's eyes staring at him, just for a split second. Then Leo smiled, and got to his feet with everyone else and left the hall. In that moment Leo felt Thomas too deeply beside him. He felt their togetherness being celebrated and accepted and protected. He felt it like a basic social right. And to defend that right a whole people would have gone to war. A whole generation would have sacrificed itself to keep their relationship intact – part and parcel of its cultural heritage. He felt bowled over by the enormity of the feeling.

While he and the other speakers enjoyed the refreshments offered by the rector, he could think of nothing else. It was a new sensation, because Leo had never before believed in the worth of acceptance. In theory, being accepted or approved of by whoever it might be did not bother him. It was inside himself that his worth and his legitimacy were lodged. Nothing to do with the outside world. And no one would ever be able to grant him that right. He existed. That was all there was to it. Only madmen wonder why they are the way they are. And yet an odd thing struck Leo in that university lecture-hall. And there was only one possible explanation: Thomas. Leo was in fact introducing himself to the outside world not as Leo, but as Leo-with-Thomas. He was no longer alone. He was with somebody else. And the world would have to take note. It would have been so simple to say: 'I love him. And everything else can go to hell.' But love needs the world to affirm itself. And Leo knew that happiness needed to stay in the world to be fulfilled. Now there was someone he could dedicate that approval to. He needed the world to take note of this new life that now existed lovingly within him.

This was why he could not sleep that night. When he started feeling down, after the official dinner, he went to their room, feeling glum and lost, and gnawed at by some inexplicable anxiety. He waited until Thomas dropped off to sleep and got out of bed. He pulled back the curtains and walked on to the balcony that ran along two sides of the room. He started pacing nervously back and forth. The hotel was built like a cylindrical tower in the middle of a large sports complex, and their room was on one of the topmost floors. Beneath him he could see the park and an artificial lake for international rowing races. There were tennis and basketball courts, jogging tracks and riding circuits. The dark shape of the stadium loomed on the horizon. At that time of night everything was still, lit by the service lights.

Thomas was asleep, dreaming, who knows? He was breathing slowly, wheezing slightly. It gave Leo a feeling of warmth and intimacy. But he felt desperate. And he did not know why. He loved Thomas. He loved him now in a way that was tormenting him. Yet none of this managed to calm him. He felt now as if he himself were at stake. Perhaps it was precisely this that scared him. There was no turning back. His life was forever bound to the life of somebody else. He should have handled it all quite differently. His stomach hurt with the anxiety about what lay ahead, hurt with the fear of the darkness that he saw all round him. What would happen tomorrow? And in a month's time? Or a year? Did they have a future? Would he be able to stand by this love? Wouldn't they both die? Wasn't everything futile? He felt his heart foundering in a surge of pity and penitence. And he lowered his head.

There was a sudden burst of light on the horizon. A dull rumble rose into the sky lighting up the area round about. It was a fiery red colour, then it turned yellow, until a glow spread right across the sky. A fire still roared at the heart of the light. Leo stayed looking at it. It was a long way off. How far he could not tell. It stayed way over on the horizon. Smoke rose into the air and then there was a second explosion, and a third. It was four in the morning. Leo went back inside, woke Thomas and took him out on to the terrace. 'It's the steelworks,' Thomas said half-asleep. Leo made him stay out there, with nothing on, in the chill night. 'You mean everything to me,'

Leo said after a moment in his shaky German, clinging to Thomas's shoulders and sobbing.

What he is really doing is running away. He is not consciously running to any particular place. He is not running to meet any particular person. There is nothing he particularly wants to do. Just the other side of the Dutch border, when he gets off the train and looks for somewhere to spend the night, he realises he is on the run. He is fleeing across Europe, fleeing from the horror of losing Thomas. He is fleeing from death. But he is running more and more slowly, more and more out of breath. He feels like some old wounded animal peeling off from the herd to look for a place to die – torn apart by wolves, wracked by disease, and withered by age. And just like an animal nearing its end, he does not want to live any more. He is fleeing from one death to draw closer to his own. He falls into a deep sleep, all afternoon and all night long. When he is not on the move, he sleeps. And each time he lies down on a bed he is sure he will never wake up again.

He keeps running northwards. He feels winter coming on, and it gives him a pleasant feeling. One day, on a ferry crossing the North Sea, fog suddenly descends without warning. All at once the sun becomes a blurred, pale disc, and then disappears. It is dark and hushed. The ship heads into the void. Leo is on the deck, astern. He cannot even see the water below. It is cold and the fog shrouds him damply. Suddenly the foghorn bellows, once and then again. An ancestral sound, like a horn urging men into battle. And to his right, a few dozen yards off, the

huge shape of a ship's hull looms through the wall of fog.
All he can see through the mist is a name painted on the
bows in Cyrillic letters. Huge white letters suspended in
the greyness that mean nothing to him. The word sails
past his eyes and suddenly vanishes, swallowed up once
more by the chill fog. He stays rooted to the spot for a
moment, then heads for the bar. He needs something
strong to drink. He is excited. He feels as if he has just
seen Moby Dick.

London was meant to have been just a point of reference, a destination. Instead, this sea crossing has turned
London into a kind of salvation. After a month of moving
from A to B, but never far, he is finally leaving the continent, and with it Thomas's tortured body. Behind him he is
leaving war, corpses, pain, concentration camps and
cities razed to the ground. England seems like a separate,
distant country, where he knows hardly anybody and
hardly anybody knows him: where he can be alone without being lonely. In England he can walk about, sit in a
pub, drink and write, and no one will look at him or
bother him. He is leaving behind him a continent that is
being destroyed. Thomas was History. His country and
his language were the scripts of war.

One night they arrived in Dresden by train from East
Berlin. The whole journey – setting out in the morning
from Kotbusser Tor, crossing the wall on foot at Check
Point Charlie, taking the East Berlin metro; reaching the
railway station – had been like a journey back through
time, what with passports and visas, declarations and
permits, and prepaid vouchers for hotels like the Karl

Marx Plaza, the Lenin Hotel and the Sozialism Palast. They had crossed Saxony by night. They had not seen a single light for more than two hours, not a single building or town. They were alone in a compartment and the light did not work. An inspector had asked to see their tickets and a policeman had asked to see their passports. Both had been extraordinarily nice, smiling and wishing them a safe journey. They had vanished into the gloom. Then the train had entered slowly beneath the great awning of the station. The lighting was dim and sallow. Hundreds of passengers, all dressed alike, men and women of all ages, scuttled hurriedly towards the exit. They all wore green anoraks and they were all carrying plastic carrier-bags, or leather briefcases and satchels, or some other kind of bundle. Leo and Thomas had stopped to look at a street plan of the city to find where their hotel was located. A little way off a silent queue of dozens of people waited in line for hot drinks which would be thrust through a small window at the end of some employee's arm. When they set off again they were completely alone, bewildered beneath the vault of the huge, desolate station.

The crowd had moved off, swallowed up by underground passages and vanishing through the exits. A patrol of Soviet soldiers came towards them. They were very young and tall, with guns, and wrapped in heavy ankle-length greatcoats. They were not like the Vopos – the East German People's Police. They were more martial, more intriguing, and more android. They were like from the past, or from a distant future. They had bright, shiny boots which clicked against the ground and disturbed the mist all around, seeming to crush and dispel it. With the light behind them, they came marching on, making the booking-hall reverberate. Thomas and Leo stopped dead. In that moment it was as if the vast station hall, the trains, the platforms, the tracks and the arrival and departure boards were all parts of a prison, or some squalid barracks, or a gigantic police station plunged into the timeless desolation of the ubiquitous pale neon lighting. The patrol marched past them, all in time together. They had a red band sewn around the coat sleeve with Cyrillic letters on it. And the star of the Red Army. Leo also noticed their gloves and even the wispy halo from the heat of their hands gripping the icy barrels of the rifles. But those soldiers did not seem to have eyes. They stared straight off into the distance, with their fur hats pulled down over their eyebrows. Speechless, Thomas and Leo turned and watched the platoon march towards the far end of the booking-hall. There, wrapped in a dark green overcoat, a porter was leaning against a rusty pillar, smoking. He glanced up at the patrol and quickly stubbed out his cigarette under the sole of his shoe. He adjusted his cap and was off in a flash. Thomas and Leo headed for the exit. They found themselves once again among a jostling crowd. Just then, without a sound, other trains had arrived, spilling out hundreds and hundreds of other passengers, all anonymous and identical, noiselessly invading the booking-hall and then forming queues for buses or walking straight out into the constructivist delta of Prager Strasse.

It was no later than five on a November afternoon and there they were closeted away in Room 904 of the

Lilienstein Hotel, watching through the net curtains the tide of commuters on Prager Strasse. There were more hotels on the other side of the street, virtually all more or less identical variations of the one module of socialist architecture. In the middle of the square stood a structure with an enormous glass dome. It looked like the set of a Godard film.

The ceiling of their room was quite low. The synthetic carpet was a sickly green. The sheets were nylon. There were two small twin beds, a sofa, a TV set that looked like a toy, and the radio selector behind the headboards. They felt as if they had ended up in a rather squeezed and oblong-shaped box, in a wide-angle photo. Everything was very horizontal. There were lightshades giving off a pale, violet light, all a bit fifties. And on the far side of the street the windows of the other hotels on Prager Strasse were lit up with precisely the same colours: mainly pink, but also orange, cyclamen and pale green.

Next day, by the river Elbe, near the city ruins, with those damaged steeples blackened by fire and those dilapidated buildings where all that remained were slender, crumbling, riblike walls, like so many mountain spurs, all Leo talked to Thomas about was his father. And the war. And as they strolled along the boulevards of the Zwinger district, a particular memory came to him, as clear as a bell. A memory that had tormented him. He was in an armchair, in his mother's arms, and they were looking at a film on TV. It was the story of a Jewish child, locked away in a concentration camp, who was saved by an American soldier. He had wept quietly, burying his face in his mother's armpit, ashamed of his tears. And at the end of the film, when his parents had turned the lights back on in the room to tidy up a bit before going to bed, he felt upset and asked them: why? Now he cannot for the life of him recall what his father or mother replied. He can just remember how a feeling of terror gripped him and ran right through him as he lay in his little bed. He was terrified. He lay all night with his eyes wide open in the dark, breathing silently so that no one would know he was there, his body curled up in fear. And he kept on thinking: 'I didn't do it. I wasn't responsible for any death camps. I wasn't even born, and I've got nothing to do with those piles of dead bodies and those ditches filled with skeletons. So why do they make me look at the gas chambers? I haven't done anything wrong. I didn't have anything to do with it. Nothing at all.'

For years and years he had been hounded by a sense of guilt over those gas chambers, over the torture and destruction, as if he, Leo the little boy, had been the person chiefly responsible for it all. Then as he grew older he managed to put it all away in a cranny of his mind. He had built a cocoon of reasons and ideologies and rationalisations around the whole thing. The cocoon did not do away with his fear altogether, but it managed to keep it in check. He had experienced moments of violence. He had seen people beating each other up in the barracks dormitory. He had seen corruption and humiliation. He had seen the strong bullying the weak, but the cocoon had never opened up. It was still there and he thought he had almost got over all that. He was grown up. He was a man now, and he knew the score.

71

Then one morning, on the banks of the Elbe, with one arm leaning lightly on his friend's shoulder, that wound of fear opened up again. And he found himself on the verge of panicking. Before he knew it, they would be coming to take him away – that is what went through his mind. They will come and take me away.

He held his head in his hands and rubbed his eyes, trying to convince himself that it was all going to be all right, that none of it was true. But soldiers drove up in a truck. Shouting and bludgeoning, they took him away from his family, from his mother and father, and he found himself alone by a gas chamber watching an endless procession of bent, desperate shadows shuffling past. In that moment he saw the war, he felt the flesh being ripped and torn, he smelt the foul stench of the crematorium ovens, and it seemed impossible to breathe the air, because the air was black and poisonous, and he could not see Thomas . . . Thomas was way, way off . . . yet the only people nearby were a few couples of elderly West German tourists, one or two American women wearing sneakers and plastic head-scarves, and a class of noisy, happy schoolgirls. And the November day was strangely clear and sunny. It was cold but everything was limpid as if inside a glasshouse. And the Zwinger gardens looked pretty and gracious – you might even say elegant. But there was something oppressive weighing on him. And all round him that language and that land terrorised him, even though Thomas was an embodiment of it, and Leo loved him.

Then they walked slowly through the galleries of the art museum, taking their time. Leo felt exhausted, as if he had just come through a fit of crying. He was shaking and his eyes could see everything with the sharpness and the sensitivity of a soul laid bare. He walked through the endless rooms and corridors that seemed to spawn yet more rooms and corridors in the large mirrors lining the walls and ceilings. He kept on seeing soldiers' arms taking down the pictures and paintings and transporting them all over Europe, rolling up the canvases, packing up the frames, and storing them all in the depths of castles to protect them from being looted and vandalised and bombed. It was as if his imagination was once again incapable of focusing on the object. Instead it latched on to the human element that had handled the object. And then he saw Prussian troops, and the armies of the Duke of Este, and the footsoldiers and mercenaries of the Central Powers, and then the Nazis and the allies and the Soviet garrisons ... and for him they had all left the imprints of their bloody, war-blackened hands on those paintings as they moved them from castle to castle and country to country amid the fires of wars. He saw those hands and those imprints and those marks stamped on the works of art. But not exactly on the figures in the paintings. Rather on the frames. On the edges. And when Leo became aware of this, he finally started to look at the paintings and managed to concentrate on what was inside the frames.

He stood motionless for several minutes in front of the large canvases where, in the background, he recognised the landscapes and cities of his native land, and not just the palaces and canals of Venice, the domes of Rome's basilicas or the mediaeval towers of Bologna. More particularly, in the works of Il Parmigianino, Carracci, Il Guercino and Dosso Dossi he saw the faces and eyes and faint smiles of people he had once known. And in Antonio Allegri's *Virgin with St Francis*, which hung originally in the church where, as a boy, he had served mass – he, the little choir-boy with his red surplice, all plump and chubby, marooned like a doll in a huge, high-backed choir-stall behind the high altar, he with his legs which did not touch the ground so he had to climb to get up into it, with the tips of his toes finding footholds among the rosettes inlaid in the friezes . . . There, in Antonio Allegri's painting he recognised the face of his catechism teacher. They were identical, the painted face and the face that he could now remember. If he tried even harder, he could even remember the teacher's name. And now he could see her in her stern and sober grey wool cardigan, with a thin gold chain around her neck, no make-up on her face, large eyes, her curly hair in a tight bun at the back of her head, and her blue skirt coming down to her calves. And the more he remembered her, the more the image in the painting took on the contours of her face, leaving the face of the Virgin Mary in the background, as if against a field of expressions and looks. And it was not just this idea of the face. It was also all those hundreds of other women's faces that had been handed down through the ages until they all took form in the final clarity of the catechism teacher's face. Because Leo was quite sure now that the model used by Allegri and the young woman in the small country chapel were related, if not by name, at least in their facial expressions and in their physical features. Together they gave form to that single face, and to that single idea which then became the idea of devotion to life: the idea of a prayer.

Then that evening they took the train back, and that journey also became relevant to the idea of revival. After a few hours they left the lights of East Berlin and crossed the wall into the noisy, corrupt traffic of the West. At around ten that night they found their way into the arty, cosmopolitan, vaguely cultural-chic atmosphere of the Paris bar. There at last, as Leo gave their order to the waiter in French, he finally felt at home, sitting down to a dozen snails and a bottle of Beaujolais nouveau. He stroked Thomas's hand as it lay on the white tablecloth, and saw the image of their hands reflected by the flame of the candle in their wine glasses. They were weary, but Leo felt happy, in every human sense of the word. He felt that among all the horrors of History there existed a point of reference for him, and he felt that he could rely on it.

It is raining when he disembarks at Folkestone. Other ships are moored at the quaysides and hundreds of people are spilling out across the wharves, running, shouting, and dragging suitcases of every shape and size. Children, girls, old West Indians, Pakistanis, students from all over the world, immigrant families arriving by train from Turkey with a collection of bundles and bags and cases and chairs. Small buses shuttle between the quayside and the customs shed. Not a hope of getting a place. Then it turns out to be even more difficult, with all his luggage, to find a place on the bus to the railway station. Leo drags his suitcases wearily along the wet, slippery tarmac of the quay. In the thick of all the confusion, with trolleys laden with parcels and suitcases and trunks constantly passing him, he cannot help feeling like a refugee. They pass containers piled high not with merchandise or food or manufactured goods, but with luggage. An enormous movement of personal belongings – clothes, socks, shirts, bars of soap, tubes of toothpaste, underwear and lingerie.

A group of women wrapped in black chadors are looking up at a crane that is moving their luggage. They have built a kind of wall on the ground, heaping one case on top of another, like so many bricks. They have barricaded themselves in behind their belongings in an attempt to build a shelter in that foreign land which will never be their country. And now they are waiting, silent and still, for the last bricks to arrive from the skies. It is already dark by the time Leo boards the train. He finds a seat in a carriage with people he recognises from the ferry or from the queue waiting to pass through customs. Two young Americans are reaching the end of their tour of Europe. They left California back in May and now it is autumn. They have travelled all round the Mediterranean, and have come back to London to catch the plane back to the United States. Their presence reassures Leo. He too can feel that he is a traveller, he can create a little make-believe for himself, see himself a few years younger than he is, travelling round Europe. He is no longer some poor fellow on the run. In a few hours he will find somewhere to spend the night, and a place to have a meal, and somewhere to spend a quiet moment.

He spends the night in a hotel near Sloane Square. He goes up to his room, opens the minibar and mixes himself a gin and tonic. He turns on the TV, runs a hot bath and lies soaking in it. At two in the morning he gets into bed and turns out the light. Beside him, in the dark, he is aware of the other half of the bed, untouched and empty. He stretches out an arm and thinks of Thomas.

Next day he starts looking for somewhere to live. He decides not to call up the few people he knows in London. The idea of being someone's guest terrifies him. He wants to be alone. He does not want to talk to anybody. Even less does he want to make dining-table conversation at seven in the evening. He does not feel like going to the cinema. He does not want to sit with a cup of tea facing two eyes wide open and trying to understand. He does not feel like having to explain himself.

He starts to do the rounds of the estate agents. Every morning he marks the places he should visit on his street map. But as the days pass his search turns into a problem with no apparent solution. He leaves the Sloane Square hotel and moves to a flat in Soho for a fortnight. He cannot stay longer, he is told, because the flat has already been booked by a couple of American professors. He can just have it until the end of the month. He agrees to the temporary let mainly to have a chance, at last, to unpack his bags.

The building is in Old Compton Street, at the Charing Cross Road end. There are stairs up to the fourth floor flat, with its two rooms, bathroom, kitchen, and a terrace. It is clean, simply furnished, and newly painted. The kitchen is fully equipped and the bathroom looks just like an Italian bathroom – not one of those freezing cubby-holes with not even a toilet he has endured before

– from St John's Wood to West Kensington to Paddington to Streatham Hill – in every London house he has ever lived in in the past.

He goes out on to the terrace. It is really part of the roof of one side of the building, covered with tar-paper and waterproofed. It is as big as the whole flat, maybe even bigger, and arranged on two levels. On one side brick steps lead up to a second smaller terrace. Here, the remains of summer are piled up and covered by a sheet of old plastic: a folding table, a few white chairs, and flower-pots with plants that are dead now. Round about there are other buildings, a couple of twenty-storey blocks, and further off the Post Office tower. In New York some-body would have turned it into a dream terrace, but the buildings in London are too low, the city is too flat, and the view for the most part is just blurred, barely visible sky.

In the nearby buildings, where the windows are lit up and curtainless, he can see dozens of people at desks, working away at computer keyboards, and sitting at type-writers. There is not a tree or a plant to be seen. He thinks how this little apartment could have been a love-nest for him and Thomas. By splitting the rent they could have lived in it for five or six months. They would have invited people round after a night at the theatre, cooked a barbe-cue, turned the stereo up full volume, and danced all night without bothering a soul. They would have strung fairy-lights and paper streamers across the terrace, corner to corner, and filled every nook with candles and flares. No, wait, they would put a spotlight right there to light up the door, a spot from a photographer's studio. Here they would put some boxes, and there the table with the drinks. What would they have prepared for their guests? Something Italian? Or a dish from Germany? No, Thomas would never have got into cooking. But he could have played the piano. They would have had a piano right here. Maybe they would not have been able to get it up the stairs. So they would have had to get it hoisted up, let's see now . . . up that way, yes, that should do it. A hired piano. Thomas will get used to it. I could invite Sara and Lisa and Paul . . . no, I don't want to see Paul. Bruno, though, if he's still in London. Then Martin and John, and, of course, David, who will bring along some trendy friend . . .

He gets up early and wanders aimlessly round Soho. He likes the city at this time of day. It is empty and quiet. The weather turns in a matter of minutes and the grey dawn drizzle suddenly gives way to a wispy sun that lengthens the shadows of the buildings and creates a crisp, dazzling chiaroscuro effect – a sequence of dark areas and light areas separated down to the last millimetre, like drawings. By nine he is already in the first estate agent's office. The employees who deal with him are surly, verging on rude. It is probably a tactic to put foreigners off. They keep telling him that there are plenty of English people looking for places to live. They mumble that he will have to be patient, and toss his application form down on the table. He smiles politely, and says a few words that no one understands. He imagines the other employees thinking that he is crazy, or at least a bit odd. The only thing he might say to explain his behaviour is 'Thomas is dying, okay?'. But he cannot bring himself to. So he does not try to explain anything. He takes the addresses they give him and wanders off into the city.

He visits houses and lodgings that he could never have imagined. For prices the equivalent of an average salary, people show him dilapidated rooms, damp, sagging ceilings, filthy little apartments with stained, smelly wall-to-wall carpets and beds and closets and kitchenettes all crammed on top of each other, and paraffin cooking rings on chests-of-drawers and minute little fridges on bedside tables. With the toilet, need one add, three flights down on the landing.

For the time being he is not interested in finding an apartment. He wants to see things and try to understand them, for Thomas's sake. He feels he has a kind of duty that is pushing him on into the most sordid boarding-houses you could ever imagine, lived in mainly by Indians, Pakistanis, African students and young Jamaicans. He feels Thomas's suffering, gangrenous body thrust close to his, so close it is stuck to his skin, nailed to him. Like some female animal dragging about the dead body of her offspring, refusing to abandon the bleeding carcass that is still warm. His pain and grief force him towards other people. Several times he jolts himself with surprise at hearing himself saying out loud in the middle of the street: 'But can't even you see the horror of it all, Thomas?'

As a student, he had seen the lodgings that are rented out to students in university cities: garrets, basements, crumbling attics where the pipes freeze up and burst in winter, corridors with campbeds where students from

Greece or Eritrea or Somalia would usually end up, sometimes even a student from the South. When he was in the army he had seen where earthquake victims lived, he had lived snowed-up under canvas in a refugee camp, he had queued in a blizzard outside the latrine trucks. And he had wondered how families could live like that for years and years. Now that he himself is a traveller with no roof over his head, he is doubly shocked by a little red-brick house squeezed between the railway tracks and the freeway somewhere behind Olympia.

There is a sort of office in the hall. The air is stuffy, reeking of closed rooms and fried food. A small Pakistani with bluish skin says good morning. They discuss the price and the formalities. Then a maid appears to show him the room. She is a fat, exuberant, red-haired woman. Her face wears an ill-tempered, mean expression. She talks in bursts as she puffs her way up the stairs. She is wearing a white shirt. Dangling down her right thigh hangs a bunch of keys and master-keys, on a large ring. Attached to each key is a small metal tag with a number or letter. The jangling noise of the keys at every step she takes is awful. Like the noise of shackles. She has a greasy red chignon on the top of her head, like a pancake, and when she lifts her leg to tackle the next step, her apron twists and slips a little on her buttocks, revealing the back of her hideously white and lumpy thigh, squeezed into a rolled down nylon stocking, like a sausage in a skin.

After the first flight of stairs they come to a very narrow passage. They walk along it, shoulders brushing the walls. At the end there is a white plywood wall with small doors like the doors of a sleeping-car. The woman selects

81

a key and pushes the door open, inwards. There are neon lights everywhere – lights that never go out. In the cubicle there is a folding bed, some rolled-up sheets, a small table covered with clothes, and an open bag with dirty laundry spilling out of it. The neon light has a sports paper rolled around it. There are no windows. A small electric cooker with a frying-pan, a few cups, and an almost empty jar of coffee. There is an unbearable stench of old food. The woman looks at Leo, and shakes her head without muttering a word. Then she flings open the doors of all the cubicles along the passage, one after the other, five or six of them. She does not knock at the doors, and she does not utter a word. She just repeats the price of the room. A young man is sprawled on a bed, wearing a foul-smelling McDonald's uniform. He does not object to the intrusion, he just covers his face with the pillow. One of the other cubicles does have a window. But it is only a quarter-size window. A tiny peephole. It is split into four quarters by the walls. That way other cubicles share it, and the cubicles on the floor above can have a window at floor level, while the cubicles on this floor enjoy a window at ceiling height.

The woman is still standing in the doorway clutching her bunch of keys. Leo says sparingly: 'Thanks for showing me. I'll let you know.' He makes to leave. He feels like taking to his heels, to forget that intrusion into the tiny, desperate intimacy of those oppressed and exploited people who work on average twelve, even fifteen hours a day just to afford those hellish tombs. He goes downstairs. On a landing he sees a row of tiny doors, almost on top of each other. He imagines what they are hiding. He opens one. In a space smaller than three feet by three are a toilet and a small washbasin. The toilet is low down and claustrophobic, like in a plane. The only difference is that here you are not flying anywhere. You are just headed for the pain and hopelessness of a life on the margins.

He has to walk for a bit to get rid of the stench of that hellhole from his nostrils. He stops in a pub for a pint. He feels like calling Italy and talking with someone. What is this decrepit old country doing to the Third World? What is this people of pirates and quarrelsome boozers doing to its former colonies and its former subjects – subjects it has oppressed with the violence of the lash after plundering and exploiting their land? What hypocrisy allows Europeans to impose their rules and their ways, as if all values still came from the West, whereas precisely the opposite is true? Why is it that from every corner of the world the most wretched souls, the poorest of the poor, the rejects of history, the hordes of down-and-outs and tramps and beggars all invade the cities where to be integrated there is nothing for it but to mimic the hypocritical selfishness of the European middle class. How can one not feel inside one a huge, deep sense of shame when you see the eyes of the Indian kid with his McDonald's jacket stretched on his bed trying to snatch a few hours of sleep between one shift and the next? The result of it all, Leo thinks to himself, is that we are all contesting with the poor – for every inch of the city. And you can already see sick old Europe, in all its splendour, with its culture and its vainglory, with its afternoon tea and its academic ceremonies, wiped out, taken over and conquered by the masses of the poorest, hungriest, most exploited poor. It will be their war. The poor will get their own back by having children wherever they go, reproducing as rapidly as a burst of machine-gun fire, taking up all the space with their own dead bodies, using their very weight to force a breakthrough. They will win in the end, and, as the gospels say, they shall inherit the earth.

Most evenings he eats in the Chinese restaurants in Gerrard Street, trying them out one by one. He insists on ordering Peking duck or duck stew, and makes a mess all over his hands and mouth and shirt. Having a meal becomes quite an ordeal. He never knows which place to choose. He wanders the streets for hours looking for a restaurant that looks just right. He walks by the same restaurant once, twice, even three or four times before deciding to go inside. He never knows what to choose from the menu and invariably resorts to the same familiar dishes every night, reeling them off by heart. Tonight a couple comes and sits beside him. Leo gets to his feet to let them squeeze past. His knee knocks the table and upsets the soy sauce. He starts to mumble an apology, smiling at the people round about as if he had offended someone. The other diners turn away, embarrassed. When he is quite sure nobody is looking he spreads his serviette over the brown stain, trying to hide it. Then he notices that the serviette has his lip marks on it, reddish and clearly visible, like blood.

One evening he is sitting in a cheap and shabby Chinese restaurant. Close by are two young German couples. The girls steal glances at him, looking inquisitive, as often happens at restaurant tables. The place is full. The owner is a tall, stiff woman in her fifties. She bustles up to his table followed by a customer, a small man wearing gloomy clothes. She pulls out the empty seat, sits the customer down and hands him a menu. Leo looks up, laying down his chopsticks. The woman acknowledges his presence for the first time, and asks if everything is to his liking. And Leo hears himself answering in an unexpectedly aggressive tone of voice: 'No. I don't like this stuff.' His words ring out through the restaurant. The Germans look at him silently. The small man looks down at the table. Embarrassment reigns for a moment. Leo blushes, but stares at the woman resolutely. She gestures to the small man to follow her, saying there is probably a better table in the other room.

This is what being single is all about, this kind of slightly comic, slightly ridiculous, slightly violent situation with a fellow at a table in a tourist restaurant – the picture of a person who is incomplete, with something missing, acting awkwardly and looking foolish or arrogant. Leo feels he must defend this aloneness. He must not let the other diners see him as some kind of anything-goes human speck, someone made miserable by the lack of a friend or a lover to eat with. Solitude can be a nuisance as well. It makes you turn to other people, and be forever asking them for things. On a train you cannot leave your baggage and go to the dining-car. You must find the inspector, or another passenger, and ask him or her to be kind enough to keep an eye on your camera. Same in airports, with a trolley full of luggage. And in restaurants people queueing for a table are forever jostling you because there are two of them and you are on your own at a small table whose location is invariably an obstacle. In hotels, single rooms are usually the meanest and the smallest – in what used to be maids' rooms, in attics and garrets. And there's invariably a supplement to add insult to injury. Solitude brings out pity in other people. Sometimes he feels people stealing glances at him, and their glances contain a repressed violence. It is as if other people regarded him as they would a blind man – someone who needs help to cross the street. Certain kinds of thoughtfulness and considerateness are more offensive than plain indifference or neglect, because it is as if he were being constantly reminded that there was something missing in him, and he can never be happy. He sees himself with one side of his body bleeding from an open wound from which the other side has been removed. He longs to explain that, yes, he does indeed miss Thomas, and that he is suffering. But on the other hand he does not feel despair at his own solitude. He is focusing in on himself, enclosing himself in his own fantasies and memories. He is trying to embrace the truest part of himself, recovering it by means of recollection and reflection and silence.

He still sleeps a lot. He sleeps in the afternoons and then turns in early. When he is lying in his single bed it is as if he is forced to recapitulate and make summaries of his past and his whole life, in order to start all over again. He hopes he will eventually emerge like a new man from this lethargy. But the more he thinks of moving on, the more he feels himself being dragged backwards.

For the first time in his life the only thing that catches his eye is children. He sees them in parks, watches them for hours playing in streets and schoolyards. As he watches, he wraps himself up tight in his woollen jacket, unable to concentrate on anything else. And he feels at peace, and gently taken outside of himself. He looks through the chainlink fences round playgrounds and schools as if he were at the zoo, or in a natural history museum. He notices how the children are dressed, how they talk, how they play and cry. He imagines them grown up. In each one of them he sees the expressions they will have when they are young and, later on, old men. He remembers other children, other schoolkids, and his own schooldays. And in all this he sees his own boyhood torment. It is an agonising feeling. It bewilders him because he can no longer get close to that chubby, tooth-less little boy, to cheer him up. He would like to lay a hand on his small shoulder and smilingly tell him there is no need to be afraid.

At such times he pulls his jacket tighter about him, hunches his shoulders and walks slowly away. The huge weight of all the violence he had to put up with as a boy feels like profanity and sacrilege – just a small vulnerable lad brimming with purity and his own naive goodness. And he feels he is going mad, because he realises that the only thing that sends you mad is acute pain. Now that small boy is slowly coming back to him. He realises that he has nothing outside of himself to fall back on. His mourning over Thomas's death, a death that is there hour by hour – how many times a day does Thomas die for him? – his mourning is crushing him. Everything inside him is breaking apart. Or rather, falling away. In silence he walks the streets, sits in pubs around Covent

Garden and orders pints of bitter, but does not talk to a soul. His English is like a child's. He spends whole afternoons playing slot-machines or video games in amusement arcades. All of a sudden, when he is in a museum, or while he is having supper, he feels an irresistible urge to plunge into the jingling, jangling space-age din of an amusement arcade where the pinball machines talk like robots, inviting you to play, and the video games play rudimentary tunes, as if they are being played by an interstellar organ, and the slot machines endlessly produce the metallic rattle of a jackpot. When he is not playing, he stands and watches. After just a few days he can pick out the regular losers, the passing tourists, the little tyrants running the arcades who always have to hand a few pounds' worth of small change so that the people playing the machines do not have to leave their machine to go and get more change, and thus abandon that probability, however remote, of a jackpot. Every now and then Leo wins too, and feels a wild thrill of pleasure which, for a split second, shakes him out of his torpor. And this thrill has nothing to do with how much he wins, it is just the sight of the winning combination coming up. In that moment he feels totally at one with the machine. You could almost say he falls in love with it. He sees himself thrust forward as a winner, and then he tries again and loses the lot.

In the arcades there are lots of orientals, and tiny Chinese women pulling at the one-arm bandits. Old men chewing on cigarettes, digging into their pockets and producing coins one by one as if each were a treasure. There are other poor wretches muttering winning oaths, and crossing their fingers, and tapping on the glass windows in front of the rotating symbols of fortune, bright and cruel at the same time: cherries, bells, pears, apricots and jokers. There are quarrels to see who will have first pull. There are frequent heated arguments, with the weakest of the two hobos finally gathering up his few belongings – often no more than a small plastic bag full of old clothes – and shuffling out cursing. In another arcade ten yards down the same street, Leo comes across the loser again, even more argumentative than before. And as he wanders aimlessly like this from arcade to arcade, or round a square or up and down a street, just for the pleasure of feeling rejected by fate and by mankind, it all reminds Leo of scoring dope.

He has been living in London for close on three weeks now. He has left the Old Compton Street flat and found a room in a small hotel a stone's throw away. It is called Hazlitt's. The rooms do not have numbers. Each room bears the name of guests who stayed there in the eighteenth century. He has been given William Duncomb's room on the top floor. It smells of wood, and has rustic pale cherrywood furnishings. There is a small fireplace where he has piled up books and newspapers. There are two armchairs and two double beds. In the morning a French girl brings him breakfast. The bread is always hot, and so are the croissants. The piping hot coffee smells wonderful. Now and then he takes a couple of cans of beer and a sandwich up to his room. He has a snack standing looking out of the window at the building opposite. In the evenings, always at the same hour, he goes to the Brief Encounter, a pub in St Martin's

Lane. There he mingles with the hundreds of men chattering and drinking – fashion models, clerks with their overnight bags on the floor between their legs, young black men, and old queens singing along together songs from *West Side Story* and *My Fair Lady*, all crowded round a grand piano. No one talks to him, and he feels fine among all those tankards of beer held aloft above his head, among those people who all seem in such good spirits, or who at least are not afraid to join in the singsong and make a noise. As ever, he watches from a corner, sitting on a stool if he is lucky enough to find a free one. Every so often his eyes meet someone else's. He turns away at once. Leo, the boy, does not like being the centre of attention or an object of curiosity.

One night he goes back to a club called Heaven. The floor is full of trendy people dancing. Upstairs, though, the atmosphere around the long bar counter is more like that of a club. He sits with a beer and watches the videos. He plays a slot machine and wins twenty pounds. He wanders all night long from floor to floor around the disco. He eats a steak and kidney pie, heated up in a microwave oven. He hears snatches of conversation. He notices how the disco crowd changes from hour to hour. When a certain group of men, all wearing fairly ordinary clothes, leaves, their place is taken first by post-punk kids with their mind-boggling hairstyles, then by a new romantic bunch, with lace-trimmed shirts, earrings, pigtails, ruffles and frills, and sailor-boy breeches. Then, last of all, the place is invaded by black men intently dancing under the amoeba-like patterns of the psychedelic lighting on the walls.

The washroom is a large room with a single urinal running all round the edge. A 'pissing wall' with its drain full of air-freshening pellets. People come in and lean against the blue-tiled wall. Leo stands in a corner. A few seconds later a young man comes and stands next to him. Leo glimpses his full, swollen sex. He sees the strong arc of urine splashing against the wall. He feels a stab of annoyance. Then anger. How can he possibly pull it out, he wonders to himself, when Thomas is dying? He buttons his fly and leaves, with the other man still standing facing the wall. He mutters to himself as he walks fast among the dancers, knocking them out of his way. He is upset, because he cannot hide the fact that it gave him some pleasure, like a spurt of energy, to realise that there are still people around who are on the make. He finds the ambivalence of his own emotional reaction absurd. He ought to kneel down and pray in the dark. He ought to go on a fast and put on sackcloth and flagellate himself with a lash. And instead he goes wandering from pub to pub, from disco to disco. He realises for the very first time that he is really not dying, as he thought. He is still alive, even if without desire. He is still alive without Thomas. Leo without Thomas. It is inconceivable. It means just one thing: Leo is dead too. Not dead in the other, who has remained faithful to the end of his life. But dead in his ideal. Because he is doomed to go on and, day after day, kill that harmonious couple called Leo-and-Thomas, that couple that is no more and will never be again. He leaves Heaven in a rush. One ridiculous encounter like that is all it takes to plunge him back into confusion and distress. He breathes deeply, as he learned to do when he was an athlete. He tries to get back in touch with himself. The night traffic on Charing Cross Road drives swiftly past, and rowdy groups of drunken revellers weave through it. No, he won't find a lover, he won't replace Thomas. As far as that is concerned he feels completely off limits. A lot of time will have to go by before he will feel ready for another affair. He has had a glimpse of a change of direction and he wants to experience it completely. Only then will he be able to find a new partner. Assuming he wants one. Assuming fate so decrees.

A few days later, on the flight back to Italy, he wonders if the journey taught him anything. He is not sure. All he knows is that since he gave up love, all he is doing is focusing in on himself. Sometimes, as he walks along a street or stands in the middle of a disco surrounded by music, or finds himself alone in his room, he hears the words: 'He's dead! He's dead! He's dead!' These words pierce his heart and his brain. He focuses on himself to learn to love the person who bears the same name as he. The person who others recognise as Leo. The person who he is finally bringing back home.

As he watches the sunset over the Alps he feels that, if he is to go on living and moving forward, he must love that same person who has had this particular seat allocated to him by the boarding-pass, this seat right here, by the window, with its view over Europe, now on the cusp between day and night.

Back home in Milan his apartment feels like an air-raid shelter. He is back among his books, and the knick-knacks he has bought from all round the world, and the candles flickering and the dozens of bottles arrayed on the mahogany table in the corner where the bar is. The city looks like a city that has just been bombed – turned inside out and torn asunder by subway construction sites, disrupted by maintenance work on water mains and telephone cables, barred by great sheets of corrugated iron protecting rusty tram-lines, riddled with holes and pits and shafts spewing up suffering, filthy men. And the smog that invariably shrouds the city seems to him like the fumes rising from rubble and ruins.

He only goes out when it is dark. He buys the next day's paper from the kiosks at Porta Venezia. He orders take-out meals and groceries by phone. People make him feel ill at ease. He feels uncertain and insecure. He often forgets to take the change at the news kiosk, or gives ridiculous tips to the errand boy from the grocery or the delivery boy from the Chinese restaurant. His cleaning-woman comes three times a week, but he does not leave his apartment. When she knocks at the door, he hides in the bathroom, and leaves her free to tidy the living room. When it is time for the bathroom to be cleaned, he locks himself in his study. And so on, through the various rooms of his apartment, making sure that he almost never bumps into her. It is as if he were fleeing, yard after yard, from beaters in a hunt whose purpose is not so much to catch him, but to flush him out by altering the layout of his lair. It feels like he is being hunted down, but he needs someone to look after him in silence.

He tries to write but is not pleased with what he writes, because, to be frank, he never manages to reach the centre of his agony and his pain. He beats about the bush, waxes sublime and ideological, but none of it satisfies him, because he knows he is still not telling the truth. He knows that he is not at one with his writing. Even though he tries different approaches and countless tactics to get closer to the core, it eludes him like the devilish target in a video game. So why write? And, most of all, why publish? Why turn this pain and grief that are so private and so essential into a small and very finite object that can end up as pulp, or ashes?

When he was not much more than a boy, he had started to write. He had gone to museums and art exhibitions. He had seen films or plays every day. All his friends talked about was football, and their improbable sexual adventures. Neither interested him in the least. The kind of life that lay behind that kind of chatter sickened him. But in the darkness of a film club or the hush of a museum he could feel his difference from others as a strength. He learnt more and more, and started to acquire knowledge. When he had started to write he did so because it struck him as the most natural way of expressing how different he felt. But now, ten or fifteen years later, even writing has become a profession for him, a craft. And when he looks at the things all around him there is a melancholy jest to his words: I earned that pair of vases from a co-editing project . . . those marble lions from India represent five reviews . . . the bed and the wardrobe a book . . . the couch and the kitchen and the bar, another book . . . and that bottle of Cognac sponsored an article on Florence. At such moments he sees everything like a prison built of words become objects of barter. The John Fante-television, the Jack Kerouac-dishwasher, the Peter

Handke-chairs, the Patricia Highsmith-plants, the Linus-table, the Rockstar-bookcase, the L'Espresso-wardrobe, the Transeuropa Editions-computer, the German translation rights-bathroom marble, the Turkish translation rights in France-rugs, the film rights-car. Words, and more words. He lives on words, eats them, quite literally. And at three or five in the morning, when he adds ice to his favourite rum in the Christopher Isherwood crystal tumbler, for a split second he wonders anxiously: 'How many words am I actually drinking now? And what story do they come from?' He had entrusted all his angst, and all his desire to change his life around, to words. Not to literature yet, not even to books, but to letters and to short stories. And now he finds himself reduced to nothing by feeling no desire either for words or for things. And if he looks beyond himself, if he sees how other people go about their lives, if he sees, above all, who exactly these other people are, these people who are involved in the same business as he, he feels once more plunged back in that high-school classroom from which he has spent years trying to escape. The others are still talking sport. So and so, they tell him, is doing well in geography, someone else in natural sciences, others in chemistry, social studies, history and religion. Among his contemporaries and colleagues, too, he sees some who have gone into academe or politics, just as, back then, he saw the fifteen-year-old son of the business consultant successfully inherit his father's practice, the chairmanship of the local Rotary Club or Lions Club, as well as becoming ward secretary of the ruling political party. He sees these careers and feels in a trap once more. He wants to quit class and leave his friends, so that he can pursue his own different destiny. But everything is harder now. There is almost no way out, because Leo is weighed down precisely by the fact that he has opted for freedom. There is no escaping now. All he can do is stay quiet and keep out of trouble.

The idea takes shape within him of writing books for ten or twenty people. Books specially written for people able to understand them, for trusted friends. He would like them to respect him and pay him some attention. He would like them not to judge whether what he has done is good or bad. Rather, he would like them to think about his readiness to take risks, and his need to relate something to somebody. He becomes obsessively jealous of what he is writing. One day, on the underground, he happens to see a stranger reading one of his books. He has to get off the train, blushing with shame. He would have liked to grab the book from the stranger's hands, hit the fellow hard and insult him. He began to walk towards him, as if obeying these very words: 'Now I'll go over and smash his face in.' Then he got off the train, confused and in a dream-like state.

When he thinks back to this incident he is struck by the idea of having been surprised, and caught with his defences down, by a total stranger. In fact he feels that that book – and other books that he has written – are like his body stripped of clothes. Not an emanation of himself, not a projection of himself, or a transference, but his actual body. Reading those pages is like getting into his very own skin, into his very own nervous system.

It is like making love with him, hating him, remembering him, and dreaming of him. This he cannot stand. Maybe, when he quit that high-school class, he really wanted all this to happen. Perhaps he wanted to serve himself up to others, by offering them a body made up of his words. Now he feels like some ageing pin-up finding a pimply kid masturbating over photos of him as a boy, and peeping lecherously in on those carnal couplings of his youth. None of this gives him any sense of narcissistic pleasure, bordering on flirtatiousness. All he has is a sense of shame and death. So if he is not writing now, and if he does not now want to write, this is perhaps not so much because he has run out of inspiration, not so much because he has lost Thomas, but rather because he is getting older. Because his body is starting to creak under the weight of everything he has already written. Basically, he is ashamed of making his body stoop with words. And so he refrains from writing and drifts back into idleness.

With each passing day he realises all the more how losing Thomas is gnawing away at him inside, with a devastating and catastrophic determination. Now he manages to sidestep Thomas's disappearance by saying to himself rationally 'That's the way it was. There's nothing I can do.' But there is no way he can repeat the same words and relate them to what is happening deep within him. For he can find no words for all this, no plausible explanations. The only thing he can do is to adopt a waiting attitude. And as he ponders this, he realises that month by month in the amusement arcades of Soho or the nightclubs of Milan, his whole life has been nothing other than a genuine and sincere prayer. For months and months everything he has done and said, or eaten and drunk, all the sleeping and travelling he has done, it has all been in Thomas's name and for Thomas's sake.

He has turned his obsession into an open gaze at himself. Since Thomas died, it is as if his sensibility has been purified. And now he is trying to head for what is essential. In this sense Thomas is not just a corpse that weighs him down, but a grain of life buried in his own mortality. Deep down, he is nurturing this grain, keeping it warm, helping it to grow, and trying to grow with it. Because with all his complicated introjections and repressions, Thomas is now the enlightened one, the one who has gone further. When Leo had seen him on his deathbed, in sweatcloths, he had thought that Thomas was changing back into Thomas-the-child; that in the short time left to him he was proceeding towards his origins; that through the enormity of his suffering he was changing not into something different, but into something that closely resembled him much more: infantile matter formed prematurely that yearned for the hush of nothingness.

So what he calls prayer is nothing more than an attitude of paying heed to things and people, observing and contemplating, and realising that he must be involved with his own way of being. He has no altars to kneel down before. He has no temples or images to offer sacrifices to. So he celebrates life itself as a liturgy. He is aware of the presence of the sacred as something tangible in reality, something on which his gaze can alight with devoutness. When he thinks of prayer he says to himself: 'I don't know how to pray. But most of all I don't know

98

who to pray to.' Then he recalls his childhood, those hours of meditation, those discussions with priests, and the recital of all those words. And in his bookcase his hand automatically seeks out the Bible. He is happiest reading the Old Testament, in particular the prophets: Isaiah, Jeremiah and Hosea. This preference is based not only on aesthetic considerations, but also, and more pertinently, on the fact that he still does not feel that redemption has arrived in his life; and the gospels appear to him like so many tableaux in a story he has yet to understand. But when he reads Hosea, when he reflects on the metaphor which makes God elect to conceive his people from the belly of a prostitute; when he considers the fact that God turns to his son in the language of a lover; when he sees him bent over the infant Israel, holding his hand as he teaches him how to walk; when he sees him enraged by the betrayal and the deaf ear with which his extreme love is returned, then Leo senses within himself his own religious calling like something that cannot be renounced. He does not have the serenity of the mystic. He simply has the inner upheavals of a soul dedicated to a quest. 'You have been bitten by the metaphysical bug,' a smiling priest friend had said to him one day.

Many a time he had caught himself saying: 'I can't live without God, but I can live without religion.' He may have abandoned the practice of religion which was part of his boyhood, and which taught him how to interpret the world, and his surroundings, and his feelings, but he did so because he would not reconcile his life and his mysticism. He did so because his quest for God was sexual as well as emotional. At the same time he saw religion being practised in a weak and mawkish way, in a way that was emasculated and enfeebled, lacking the fertile passion and the violent receptivity of femininity or the exuberance of virility. A religion without sex for people who are afraid of the passions and the power of love. An accommodating, bourgeois religion, that is more often than not hypocritical. At the same time, on the other hand, even in his silent prayers, he was aware of putting his entire sexuality on the line. This is why he read Hosea. Because in those pages there was not an exclusively mental or spiritual vision of the relationship between God and His people. Rather, there was a representation of bodies, a representation of prostitution and wantonness, of the frenzy of separation, of wrath and of paternal protection. As has always been the case since time immemorial between people who love one another.

At times he had prayed while he was making love. His eyes strayed over the naked object of his desire with a most chaste, even virginal, reverence. He was aware of the miracle of having beside him the beauty of creation, and the wonder of being able to gaze upon it in silence. The wonder of being able to touch it with the rapt tips of his fingers, just as his eyes could stroke mountains at sunset. There was not the remotest notion of possessing the other, or having dominion over him. He did not want to steal anything, claim anything, or take anything away. He wanted everything to stay intact as it was in a feeling of gratitude and fullness. Hours could pass by in these insightful moments in which the loved one's body became the universe, with its various constellations and its various worlds. And those occasions when it was Thomas who became immersed with him, whose eyes and hands ran across his body, on those occasions he would also pray, slipping off into slumber, because he was feeling the joy of experiencing his embarrassing finiteness as something that gave peace to others. He had used up most of a lifetime to achieve these moments of love and devotion – because they were in reality occasions to take stock – and from Isaiah and Virgil he called them the Golden Age. They were moments of such intimacy that some instinctive modesty had prevented him from ever talking about them with Thomas.

The desire for religion was triggered off when Hermann left him. In that period the sense of separation made Leo feel that he was constantly reduced to nothing. He felt he could not live without some values that were strong and comforting. In that moment he resurrected religion from his own consciousness, saying to himself: 'If I've been a believer for eighteen years, why can't I go on being a believer?' But he really did not manage to go on. He had gone to see a priest and he had told him, under the confessional oath, what was happening to him. As he spoke, embarrassed and confused, he realised that the person who was most perplexed was in fact the priest, who stammered 'My God! My God!', while clutching his rosary. Leo could see the sweat running down his fingers that gripped the rosary. And then with a gesture of pride, because nothing gives one more courage than seeing others in a state of confusion and embarrassment, he, Leo the man, had said to the priest: 'I want to live the way I am. Why should my freedom be judged by the conscience of others? Why should I be reproached for things for which I give thanks? This is written in the first epistle to the Corinthians. So why should I repent? I want to be happy. The fact that I must live seems atonement enough in my eyes. Only one man has been saved, father, not ten, or a hundred, or a thousand. And if one life was enough, just one, to reconcile a billion creatures to God, then this can only show us the huge pain of living. I cannot love the religion of sackcloth and suffering. I would like to love the religion of fullness. I want to be happy in my religion, because I experience it like a biological need, like eating and drinking and making love. But you don't seem to understand this. I'm trying to tell you all this sincerely, but you deny my very existence. Yet for all you and I know, even dogs have a God.'

No, in this way it was just a trap. He could have joined a religious community. They would have been delighted to take him in. They would have felt even more in the right because the lost sheep had returned to the fold. But he could not give up his very own self. He could not cripple himself, and become one of those millions who are emasculated by religion – a poor, soul, dejected and penitent, and impoverished by the world. And for this reason he had slowly, day by day, aborted his need for God. If the fact of Hermann leaving him high and dry had pushed him towards a solitary pilgrimage and introspection, his separation from Thomas is pushing him towards religiousness and the sacred. With Hermann, perhaps, he had fully realised his need for the flesh-and-blood absolute in a love affair. And when he had been robbed of that, he had sought out in compensation the experience of mysticism. With Thomas he had built up their relationship in quite a different way. There was no difference between the degrees of love he had known with both of them, because love, like pain, can neither grow nor diminish. But there was a different angle with Thomas. From the outset he knew that Thomas would never be 'everything' to him. This is why he called their love 'separate rooms'. He experienced being with Thomas in the intimate knowledge that they would split up sooner or later. Separation was an essential strength in their relationship, and an essential part of it too, just like the idea of attraction, or growth, or sexual desire. It represented an awareness that if you did not stop the other person from leaving, this made the relationship all the more human. With Hermann he had never felt death so close to his love. With Thomas he felt only death in relation to life.

Hermann, so very handsome, had come into his life one day in a museum of modern art. Leo had caught a glimpse of him at the far end of a gallery, on his own, looking at a painting close to and then drawing back from the wall to get a different perspective. He was very tall, with a slight stoop, and a lock of blonde hair that fell over an angular face. Leo did not know Hermann from Adam. But he fell in love with him. He thought he had ended up with a Chez Maxim's, but instead he found himself spending two years with a 'wrong blonde'. It was not that Hermann did not love him, but the fact was that Leo experienced their relationship as hellish. Moments of agonising neglect, tears, hugs to make up and then days of violence, separations, infidelity and betrayals.

Hermann came and went from Leo's apartment without any fixed schedule. He would vanish and resurface, sometimes in the dead of night. And Leo had to put up with all his craziness. But he still found Hermann terribly beautiful, and when Hermann nestled in his arms Leo felt jolted right down to his innermost depths by the love he bore him.

One night, in Rome, Hermann came home bleeding and covered in bruises, with his shirt ripped and a broken tooth. It was summer, a sweltering, baking hot July, and they were living in a room at the end of Via del Serpente, in the Suburra district. It was a small, windowless room, where the double bed took up almost all the space. The walls were made of plyboard, flimsy and covered in damp stains. They could hear their neighbours shouting and screaming, the noise of a man coming back home at night drunk, of children shrieking, of a desperate woman. There was a small bathroom with a toilet and a shower. The drain was blocked and you had to be careful not to use too much water when you washed, otherwise the whole room would flood. This happened every time Hermann had a shower. He would emerge grinning, pretending to swim. Newspapers floated on the wall-to-wall carpet and Leo felt desperate. Then Hermann would fling himself on top of him and he was incapable of pushing him away.

Leo was meant to be working on a film production. But he could not get into the swing of things. He was often late for meetings, and there were no ideas in his head. He would keep in touch with the director by phone, from a booth on Via Nazionale. If the line went dead he would often be out of tokens, and then he did not know how to get back in touch with him. One day, while he was talking with the production office, he smelt something burning and suddenly the phone-booth was filled with smoke. He stumbled outside leaving the receiver hanging there. Hermann was sitting on the pavement holding a box of matches. He had set fire to the telephone directory, just for something to do. And Leo had not turned on him. Instead he had burst out laughing and they had hugged and kissed and crossed Via Nazionale bringing the traffic there to a standstill, banging on the bonnets of cars just inches away from them, whistling and swearing like two happy hooligans.

Anyway, that night in Rome, Hermann had come back covered in blood. The pushers had dropped out of sight, and dealing was happening in holiday resorts. The few junkies still in town were coming in from the suburbs and preying on other desperate souls, physically attacking them to steal a fix. It was a war between human rejects, between wild animals. Hermann had been mugged in a small park, trying to score some heroin. The very same people who had been with him the night before had attacked him, beaten him up and taken the wretched stuff that he was filling himself with. He had gone back home a wreck. He sobbed and suffered. He begged like a kid who wants food. So Leo went out, cruised the square, went to a couple of bars behind Piazza Navona, eventually struck a deal, waited for hours and hours on the outskirts of Trastevere surrounded by whores propositioning him – and all he could muster up by way of response was a few angry words. The dealer finally came back, gave him the dime bag, and Leo hurried home.

Hermann was lying prostrate on the bed. He had thrown up. A bottle of brandy had spilt on the floor, and rolled into a corner. He had lit dozens of candles and the smell was unbearable. He had burnt a newspaper, page by page and black ash was everywhere. The heat was like a crematorium. Leo told him he had found a fix. He tossed it on to the bed and went and sat on the lavatory. For almost an hour he did not hear a sound. Then he saw Hermann coming towards him completely naked, with that innocent, bewildered look he had when he was high.

Hermann knelt at his feet and kissed him, clutching his legs. He had undressed him, and licked the tears that sprang silently from Leo's eyes. Hermann had asked Leo to forgive him and had given himself up to Leo's embrace with a fearful tenderness, guiding his hands, inviting him and exciting him. Leo had made love in tears. Once more he had managed to take his revenge against that love of his, hitting and beating it, and sapping it in the fury of their embrace. And he felt devastated because he saw what he considered to be the most beautiful thing in the world, Hermann, subjecting himself to the most ferocious brutality. He saw beauty being hurt and it made him feel mad. If there was a place somewhere for Hermann, it could only be among the Archangels. Instead he had tumbled into the pain of the world, like an angel that was damned. And Leo's love, and everything Leo was capable of doing for him, to the point of sacrificing his own life – in fact what he was in the process of doing – all that was doing was causing them more and more harm.

He had realised that for Hermann he was becoming a sort of necessary torturer. Someone who would not tear Hermann away from his own destruction, precisely because he loved him. And this myth, that Leo had lived for years in the sluggishness of life in the provinces, was exploding within him with a fury that he would never have believed possible. They were just two young men sprinting towards their own destruction with a determination that knew no obstacles. They were two beautiful people who revelled in being hurt and attacked because they both reckoned that the world did not deserve them, and they reckoned there was nobody to understand their qualities. They were at war with the values of society, and at war against normality. They were rebels, and they felt different. Their relationship, in a nutshell, was a war.

But as time showed with the relentless passage of the years, they were really just two young people caught up in a kind of insane escapade. This escapade would have the effect of getting rid of all their friends, one after the other, and thus wiping out those they saw as the most brilliant of their generation. Year in year out they would watch their contemporaries, twenty-seven years old, twenty-eight, thirty, thirty-two, die. Die from overdoses, from alcohol, from heart attacks, from heart failures, and murder. And just when life finally seemed to have got the upper hand, with marriages, and promising careers, and good jobs, that is when the past would come back to haunt you, one day, or one night, or on a journey. The past would hit back with the fatality of a blow below the belt.

One January night, in Florence, Leo had decided to leave Hermann. He could not carry on one more day with this obsessive feeling that had been slowly killing him for years. There were only two feasible solutions: they must either both die, or they must split up. And Leo wanted to live. So when Hermann left the apartment at three in the morning, after one of their frequent rows, Leo had taken the photo of Hermann he had been carrying for years in his wallet and thrown it in the dustbin. For months he had been trying to do this very thing, but courage had always failed him. Looking at a bin full of garbage, he would invariably put the photo back in his wallet. That night, or rather that morning, with unusual composure and an ease which surprised him, he managed to do it. All of a sudden he felt a weight off his shoulders. He breathed deeply and went back to bed, saying to himself: 'I've done it, I've done it!' From that moment on, suffering like only a person forsaken can suffer — because he had been abandoned and the fact that the decision to call it a day had been taken by him, and him alone, was really only a way of making clear a situation that had been dragging on too long: that things with Hermann could not go on — from that moment on Leo never looked for him again. And when their paths crossed, years later, in a house by the sea, he was sure that he had gone on loving him and, at the same time, that such a thing was not possible. Not in this life, nor in any other.

If he thinks back to Hermann now, to that parting, and links him inevitably to losing Thomas, he realises that after that first relationship he had clung on to a desire to

108

find someone for himself, a desire to put his own life back on the right track. And lo and behold, Thomas came into his life, after a few minor adventures on the side. But now Thomas's disappearance put him back to square one in his search for a new partner. Hermann had thrown him into Thomas's arms. Thomas's death leaves him completely alone, with no desire to start all over again. If anything, as the days go by, his death leaves him with a terror, nothing less than a physical fear, of having to start all over again with someone else. Thomas's death is shattering the karma of love's reincarnations. Leo is starting more and more to think, or delude himself, that he will only ever find safety in this new solitude. He will not give up life, just pain. And in the name of some higher value – his own survival, no less – he will do without love and sexuality.

In this way losing Thomas is carrying him along on the long path towards himself. Now that Thomas is dead and has turned into a presence vibrating and living within him, the greatest effort of his life involves accepting the discovery of his own solitude. This is why he decides, one windy day in March, to go back to the town where he was born, back to the house he lived in for twenty years, under the same roof that protects his parents as they sleep.

A small town in the lower Po valley. It has colonnades, cobblestones on the main thoroughfare, a church consecrated to the town's patron saint, a Renaissance palace, towers and belfries, a castle, an old quarter with nineteenth-century houses, and one or two eighteenth-century mansions. The fabric of the town is still intact, gathered about the old city walls now in ruins. Leo was born here in a large, old house looking out on to the main square. It is still there, but not for much longer. It has been abandoned. The tenants have gone, and with the exception of the barber all the storekeepers on the ground-floor have abandoned their shops. Demolition work will start before long, and the town will be given another building with neither history nor style.

A building filled with one- or two-room apartments, low ceilings, faceless windows, and post-modern in salmon-pink or bluish-green plasterwork. But he is not shocked. His parents would see things in exactly the same way. Only prisoners need space. And city-dweller Leo would keep everything as it is, with his reverence for the past. He is dumbfounded, for example, that a small devotional chapel, built in the nineteenth century, and still standing on the main road just a few yards from his birthplace, should have been left in a state of total neglect.

When he was a boy, Leo's grandmother would walk him in front of this little church, take him by the arm and show him the altar inside, with the painting of the Virgin Mary and the vases of flowers. For many of the townsfolk there is a tree that records the changes and developments, and the passage of time. Many of them remember that that sixty-five foot fir tree was planted by their father when they were children. Leo also recalls planting the poplars, tall now, in front of the high school buildings one October day that had been dedicated to trees. But he feels nothing when he sees that line of poplars. Not so when he walks past the chapel in the street. It reminds him of when he was a boy, and had to clamber up the iron

grille to see inside. Now he can see inside with no trouble. He is taller. And the chapel has grown smaller, more
huddled, and its outline is sharper. It is possible that the
chapel is more alone too. But for him it is still a way of
measuring time.

He parks his car on the tree-lined boulevard, not far
from the chapel. He notices that they have put two metal
rubbish bins close by it, and one side of the chapel is
covered with flyers and posters. It makes him realise that
his sense of preserving reality, or rather preserving what
he has known, or been fond of, is very different to other
people's sensibilities. He is quite sure that if he were to
ask his fellow citizens – all several thousand of them –
where he might find a certain chapel, built in a certain
style, with a particular religious painting inside, and
vases of flowers and a rusty grille with the initials of the
Virgin Mary, nobody would be able to tell him. Maybe
not even his own mother. He realises that the way he is
able to see and perceive the town where he was born is
radically different. He remembers it with affection,
tempered now by distance and detachment.

When the house he was born in has vanished, when the
chapel he clambered to see inside has been demolished,
when all the old stones have gone, it is not only the
memory of the people he loved in his childhood that will
die, it is he himself who will die as well. The next generation will not know anything about these small people
who have punctuated the history of the place – people
who will leave no trace, people whom nobody will
remember. Humble, anonymous folk, but people he felt
at one with, people who in a certain sense embraced him,

just as they embrace the whole future. When the little chapel stands in ruins, which is undoubtedly what will happen to it, he will feel even more alone. And without noticing a thing, the town will lose another small, infinitesimal fraction of its sensibility.

The cemetery stands on the far side of the house his parents now live in, which, in turn, stands right opposite the house where he was born – the house his family left more than twenty-five years ago. At the end of the boulevard, a mile or so away, the road makes a sweeping bend where it joins the new ringroad. This is where the cemetery is, close by the municipal water-tower. No matter how much Leo has travelled the world, no matter how many places he has lived in, or will live in across the length and breadth of Europe, his whole life will be contained in this walk that leads from his birthplace to the graveyard. A mile or so that he will walk down like the stations of the cross, along a path of incarnation and suffering. 'Here and yonder' is a mental attitude that he now repeats as he looks along the boulevard and then back to the windows that gave him the first view of his life. 'Here and yonder' sums up his whole life.

His mother is waving to him from the balcony. She has spied him standing still in the middle of the roadway and called out to him in her shrill voice, the voice of a young country girl, that has not changed from one decade to the next. She is still that lass who used to run through fields shouting, calling out to her sisters through the rooms of the large farmhouse where she was born. When these other women get together, they also use the same gestures and make the same din that they made in their far distant communal youth. Four sisters parted by marriages and the different towns and cities where life had led them, into small apartments where they yelled from one room to the next as if they were still in the country.

When the four of them get together, in a bedroom before Sunday mass, and parade in front of the mirror, and perfume themselves and adjust each other's clothes and the bows on their blouses and their head-scarves, chattering excitedly all the while, about who has had a house built, and who has died, and who has been unfaithful to whose wife, and who has been elected to the town council, and gossiping about trains and buses, grape-harvests and grandchildren, Leo watches them in awe, standing in a corner, feeling a sense of complicity. He would like to be invisible so that he could watch them more closely. He would like to record the interwoven strands of their chatter – as, indeed, he had secretly done now and then – the way they speak, their little shrieks, their cursing, their huffing and puffing, and those signs of the cross that they each make so swiftly, like spells. He sees how hierarchy and seniority are mirrored in their group. He notices the coalitions that are struck up between the two youngest and the two oldest. Or the sudden alliances whereby one sister is suddenly ostracised by the other three. And all of it happening in a whirligig of high heels, furs, mothballs, face-powder, earrings, and foundation creams that none of them, past sixty, has ever learned to apply without exaggeration. And all of them yelling and shouting in their rapid, shrill dialect, with each one trying to outdo the others. The end result: a babble made up of gestures, and sisters darting to and fro across the room, and laughter in front of the mirrors, and sudden lulls – a stampede, in a word, such as probably went on in their own house on Sunday mornings, before they all stepped up into the carriage to go off to mass in the village church. And when he sees them filing out one after the other, each one of them closing and reclosing the doors, with much slamming and flapping of doors and windows and shutters, because none of them trusts any of the others to close up properly, so they each open and close everything all over again with a fine sneer of self-satisfaction and spite, then Leo joins the end of the line, quiet and a little hunched, quite sure that the people who hold the reins of power on this earth are not men, but women. He sees these ladies, who are well past sixty, still showing all the vigour of young girls. He has seen them bury their husbands and withstand the slings and arrows of time, never, never ill in hospital, but always ready to assist their recuperating menfolk suffering from the frailty of their sickly bodies.

When he imagines his mother walking through the colonnades in the town, wrapped in her fine fur coat, with grandma's gold earrings and always just a bit too much make-up and face-powder, or when he hears her 'amens' rise up through the church as if she were back in the days of her childhood, he experiences a split second of terror. He prays that a chicken will not start strutting down the middle of the nave, or that a pheasant will not run across the main aisle, because if such a thing happened he would see her throwing down her fur coat, hoisting up her skirts, pulling off her orthopaedic shoes, and chasing the hen through the churchgoers, yelling and clapping her hands until she had caught it. And once she had grabbed it, she would wring its neck with a broad smile across her face, or snap its spine with a swift twist of the head. Then she would return to the congregation in church, or the crowd in the square, proudly displaying her trophy. When he finds his mother in a crowd of people he always has this same feeling of dread, and he looks anxiously and nervously about him, checking to see if there is not some poor unsuspecting chicken near at hand. Because despite all the years that have passed, he still sees his mother as a young and frisky peasant girl. And when he imagines her, thousands of miles away, trying to clutch at the image of her, he always describes her to himself with the same words, just to remind himself: 'Like a poor, everlasting, most beautiful Jewess.'

Now she comes towards him by the lift. She hurries to take his bags before she even says hello. He steps back abruptly: 'Let me take them, mama.'

They go up to the apartment. It is dark, with just the bluish light from the television to lighten the gloom in the living-room. His father is stretched out in an armchair fiddling with the remote control in an endless search for thrillers and mini-series. They say an awkward hello to each other, with that alien feeling that comes from their mutual awareness that their lives are so very different. His father gets to his feet and turns on the light. Leo makes to stop him, not wanting to disturb him.

In the kitchen one half of the table is laid with a small clean tablecloth. There is a bottle of red wine to open and a bowl of salad. His mother heats up the stew. They both eye each other without a word passing between them.

115

Next door the room resounds with gunshots and screeching police cars. Leo runs a hand through his hair, wondering if his mother is thinking he is much balder than the last time she saw him. Then he notices her adjusting her skirt, straightening it at the sides with a quick unconvincingly absent-minded gesture. Maybe she is wondering if Leo has noticed that she has put on a little weight. At the same moment they both look up, and their eyes meet, and they ask each other: 'How are things?'

Leo adds quickly: 'I'm not that hungry, mama.' Then he regrets his words, because now he will trigger off his mother's reaction about all that muck that people cook the world over and how he will always eat his fill in restaurants, not to mention that insult, that sacrilege – Chinese cooking. I've seen those Chinese people, where your father works. A boiled fish and a couple of pounds of rice, all mixed up and cooked together, guts, blood, onion, rosemary, the whole lot in the same pot, just like during the war, and then they all eat from the same pot with their hands. Go to your restaurant, go on with you.

Leo smiles because what he really cannot digest any more is his mother's cooking – the food from his own land. But he does not let on. He pours a glass of wine and drinks it down in one gulp. He will always have fond memories of this fresh, aromatic wine.

His father is a man who has not been successful in his life. He has not made much money. He does not talk much. He still gets up at dawn to go hunting in the Apennines. Or beating in the countryside nearby with his dog. The most recent thing he has done, as far as anyone knows, is to build a small bird pen around a natural

116

spring, out in the country. Every day he prepares the feed for the fish and the birds – ducks, peacocks, pheasants and chickens. An Egyptian friend has given him a pair of pink flamingoes, and they are managing to survive in what he stubbornly calls his oasis. He wants them to mate and reproduce and start a colony. Every now and then, with his friends and their wives, they organise fishing competitions, or they wring the necks of a dozen chickens and cook them in a prefabricated shed. They will spend a whole Sunday there, from dawn until dusk.

The women knead dough and fry dumplings. The men besport themselves angling for handsome pike, catfish and perch. Among their friends, with every passing month, there are always more widows or women who have lost their lifelong companion. But there is nothing sad about their gatherings out at the oasis.

It is just some overgrown pond gone wild with a few fish and a few animals, but Leo feels that his father really loves the spot. It is his private paradise, a place where he can do what the hell he likes. It probably reminds him of his own childhood and his life in the country. It reminds him of his solitude. Leo appreciates this solitary, unsociable side of his father's character. He feels the same. They are two men who have not communicated with one another, or had any physical contact with one another for at least twenty years. They avoid each other. They certainly do not seek each other out. And they ask absolutely nothing of each other. One mirrors the other, and Leo is well aware of this. He wonders if his father is aware of it, too.

After supper he chats with his mother in the kitchen. To stop her asking questions, he asks her what has been happening in the town, who has got married, who has been burgled, who has got divorced and who has given birth. All it takes is one small question to set his mother off telling him about the whole world and his wife, darting pell-mell from one story to the next. He laughs and chuckles and surreptitiously pours himself more wine until his mother whisks the bottle off the table, still chattering, and still fixing him with her slightly severe gaze. The news she gives him is comforting. Even when they talk of friends ailing with cancer and close to death, and his mother sniffs and wipes an eye with the hem of her apron, with a shake of the head, Leo finds nothing 'tragic' about it. It is as if it were all part and parcel of town life. Birth, death, people parting, they are all just stages in the collective life of the place. This life always leaves room for hope, because the community survives and evolves. Everyone leaves children and friends and fond memories behind, and the life of the town carries on an inch at a time, founded on these deep-seated bonds and feelings. Leo understands his mother's suffering, or her enthusiasm when she recounts a journey with aunts and friends and describes the cabins on the ferryboat as if Leo had never seen such a thing, or the lounges of some Grand Hotel, as if he had never set foot inside such a place. He understands but he does not feel either anguish or happiness. It is all part of a life that is not his, a life in which he will never find a foothold. All he can do is listen, smile and feel melancholy. In his body he can never feel the state of good or evil in the life of the people of his town. He enjoys watching his mother. He enjoys her stories which make him laugh until he cries. But it is all just at

118

some slight remove from him. It is as if he is a witness to life in a town apart.

When his thoughts revert to his own tragedy, he feels horror and despair once again. Because he knows that it is a drama that belongs to him, and to him alone. He knows that, in the years to come, no one will remember his lost love, no one will rest a hand on his shoulder to tell him it will all pass. He will not show his mourning on the main street of his own home town. He will not see other people's eyes reflecting the pain that fills his. He will not shake hands or embrace anyone else. And no one will accompany Thomas's body to the cemetery, not even he. He realises that this, too, is part of a separate town. A different world, in fact, which lives and suffers and rejoices parallel to the other one. He knows that the hardest thing for people is to achieve some contact with the world of other people. Going out and meeting other people with sincerity. Leo tries to blend these two remote and different worlds. But it seems impossible. He does everything possible knowing that it will be quite useless. It is just possible that things might change in the future, but many years hence. People will be born who will try other ways of combining the different worlds in which people go on living. Eventually, someone will come along for whom the memory of 'Leo-and-Thomas' will be accepted and guarded as something life-giving and hopeful. But only in years to come. Maybe not for centuries. In some ways the room which was his for twenty years is no longer the same. It is still a bedroom, with the same old bed, the same white writing-table and the same shelves fixed to the walls full of paperbacks and schoolbooks and university textbooks. But it is still not the same. It does not have him, Leo, between these four walls. All that remains now is wistful reminders or meaningless vestiges of the past, all lifeless now.

It is like reading manuscripts in the showcases of a museum. Publicity posters for sneakers, Levi jeans, pirate radio stations like Central City Radio and Anti-Radio Rock Station and World Radio are still stuck to the door, along with signs saying 'Marijuana Right On' and 'Nuclear Power No Thanks', the blue-green emblem of the Superski season-ticket in the Dolomites, the yellow mouse of 'Aktiv gegen Berufsverbote!', the WWF panda. The blow-up of a black-and-white photo of him still hangs above the stereo, where his old albums of Leonard Cohen, Nina Simone, Tim Buckley, Cat Stevens, and Neil Young are all mixed up with his mother's records of Edith Piaf and Luciano Pavarotti. A piece of dark wooden furniture in a corner contains a sewing machine. A large ironing-board leans up against the wardrobe. And beneath the desk there is a vacuum cleaner.

His room has been invaded by household gadgets. And it has changed. Every time he has come back home he has noticed his things differently arranged, until they finally vanish altogether. His large film posters of *Cabaret* and *Straw Dogs* are no longer around, probably thrown into the wastepaper basket. The photos of the Italian Film Festival of 1973 have gone, and so have the photos of his friends. The photos of Claes Oldenburg and Yves Klein, once pinned to a cork board behind the bed have also gone. The walls have changed colour as well. They used to be a very light, almost a transparent green. Now they are bright yellow.

His room has turned into a sort of boxroom. It is in this room, which looks more and more like a broom closet, he wrote his first words, his diaries, the essays for his degree, and his very first book. While he wrote, he stared out from that balcony at the town lights twinkling beneath the distant peaks of the Apennines. Out there, that was where life was really happening, and in the wretchedness of his boyhood, here up on the eighth floor, all he could do was dream about it and describe it. Imagine it like a maelstrom of people dancing from one bar to the next, and from parties to discos. Describe it like a city of night where dreams sparkle and where everyone is merry and dressed to the nines and beguiling in their cars speeding across the plain. He sits down now at the table, where he always used to sit. He has to move the steam iron and a bottle of distilled water to see out through the window. But he cannot see anything. He tries to lift up the heavy wooden shutter, but to no avail. It gets stuck halfway, askew like a guillotine blade.

The books he left behind last time are still on the bedside table. He only ever manages to read them here in this room. Books by Antonio Delfini and Silvio D'Arzo. From the balcony of his room he can see where they were born, just a few miles away. It is only in their books that he finds those particular types of madness, boredom and melancholy that are not normally associated with the people from his native land. But he is tired of descriptions of a lively, open, jovial and sensual people. What interests him now is the hidden side of this character, the dark side that causes suicides, creates rifts, and makes village idiots. It is only in these two writers, in their different ways, that he finds descriptions of that particular impenetrability of the Emilian character, that particular offhandedness, that eccentric, mad melancholy that he has known in his father and now sees in himself. He undresses and slips into bed. He opens one of Delfini's books and starts to read:

'If we had ever had the gift of lamentation and ill-will, despair and dogged hope, the expectation of bitterness and the impossible relinquishment of love dispersed, in the midst of the world's disasters and the remorseless march of time or the march of man; we would say . . .'

It occurs to him that, once again, he has gone to bed early, as he had done for a long time.

Holy Week is drawing near. The town is getting ready to experience it in a spirit of togetherness, as it does for the Christmas and New Year's Eve festivities, for All Souls' Day and for All Saints' Day, and for every ordinary Sunday. In every home and in every family, people are getting ready to do the same things, regardless of their social and cultural status. The passage of the seasons is punctuated by such activities as the grape-harvest, January pruning, bottling the new wine, and the summer harvests of sweet-corn and beet. In October, carts laden with grapes block the roads leading to the town. There are long queues of cars. From their tractors, farmers double as traffic police-men, waving cars past, pointing to a way round. Beneath the colonnades, in the bars, and at café tables, the only topic of conversation for schoolmaster, shopkeeper, or labourer, is whether the wine will be better or worse than last year. At midday on the first of the year the town is deserted, and were you to walk along the main street you would hear the popping of bottles being uncorked. Behind the window-panes, misted over from the warmth of food, you would glimpse an old man holding a grandchild in his arms, a girl smoking a cigarette, an elderly, red-faced lady loosening her blouse and fanning herself with a white serviette. On Christmas Eve families gather for the traditional meatless meal of pumpkin pie and marinated fish. Leo's favourite is eel. He only ate eel at this time of year. He leaves the large eel for his father, and the salmon for his mother. He smells the aromas of his childhood, or at least the odours of the Christmas Eve supper-table. He does not want to move on, he does not want to become something better. Everything pushes him backwards, towards his family traditions. So even the scorched little eel on his plate becomes a symbol. Why? Because since Thomas died all he has to live off is symbols.

On Good Friday the whole town gathers around the church for the procession of Christ Crucified. All morning women hang purple and black mourning cloths from the houses that give on to the main street. If you walk through the narrow alleys of the old town centre you can sense an atmosphere of sorrow. In fact what the town is getting ready for is nothing other than a funeral procession. There is nothing folkloric about it, there is no element of festivity. Everything is mournful, excruciatingly so.

After a trip to the South of France by car, Leo and Thomas had headed south across the Pyrenees, ending up in

Barcelona on Good Friday. They stayed in the Hotel Montecarlo, near the Plaza de Catalunya. The little balcony of their room looked out on to the chestnut trees of Las Ramblas. More precisely, it looked straight down on an aviary full of exotic birds. Beside the aviary were dozens of small cages with canaries, doves, blackbirds, jays, peacocks, hens and pheasants. The chirruping of the birds was like a shrill medley. As soon as the canaries hushed, the parrots chimed in, and after the parrots, the crows. It was all part of the life of Las Ramblas, together with the yelling of drunks by night, police sirens, the sharp crack of bottles hurled out of speeding cars, and the loud propositions of the prostitutes on the far side of the boulevard.

Thomas did not know Barcelona. He had never been in Spain. He walked around the city as if he were hypnotised, following Leo and tugging at his arm. At times he would stand for ages at a market stall, counting the types of olives in their large jars – every shape and colour under the sun, black, orange, purple, dark green, light green, small, large, oval and round. Or he would stand gazing at the jute sacks brimming with hot peppers in a colonial-style grocery. It was a small shop full of sacks and bags containing every manner of spice and pepper and chillies and saffron. The colours were totally pure, like powders for mixing paints. The air smelt of flour, as if it were made of fine, pepper-dust that tickled the nose and the mouth. The harsh, strong smell was almost more than they could bear. The assistant did not seem to want to be bothered with them. He was wearing a white shirt with black satin over-sleeves. He wore a small cap and metal-framed glasses. A shaft of sunlight filtered through the window and beamed through the dust from all the spices. Leo and Thomas did not ask for anything. They stood there looking about them at the sacks from Brazil, India and Africa. When they left the shop, noses sniffing and tears in their eyes, they were in a great mood, and felt the need for a sangria.

The sun was already hot, although it was still early morning. They sat down at one of the cafés in the Plaza Real, looking up at the tall palm trees. Leo idly rolled a cigarette.

A few freaks were lounging by a fountain in bright-coloured trousers, with long hair, guitars, waistcoats and broad-brimmed pale leather hats. A few men were ambling round the square offering hashish. They gathered a small handful of young men around them, sold a few joints, and then moved on as if they were playing some court game. The symmetry of the square was just like a theatre. Here, though, there was also the fascination of modern architecture, and an intense heat. The long, tall blinds on the mansions were open. Leo imagined a black-haired girl with bare shoulders coming to the window. And the colours of his fantasy were red and black and white. Leo touched Thomas's arm to say something. And he saw his bare torso relaxing in the chair, legs apart, eyes closed and tilted up towards the sun. He felt like kissing him, but was happier caressing him with his gaze. He noticed the glisten of a bead of sweat running from his armpit. Leo stared at him, filled with desire.

Suddenly the square echoed with running footsteps and the sounds of a group of children. Thomas opened his eyes and looked about him in bewilderment. Leo pointed at the children. There were a dozen or so young Nazarenes wearing tunics and cloaks. Some of their heads were bare, others wore cone-shaped hoods with slits. As they ran their cloaks filled like sails. They were barefoot and carried large candles. They crossed the square shouting and waving their arms. A group of kids tagged along behind them mimicking their litanies, a chorus of taunts and insults and whoops of joy. The Nazarenes passed a few yards from them and Leo watched those young, statuesque feet, all clean and long like an embodiment of tension itself, thrusting against the cobblestones and then suddenly flying forward as they ran on. Some of them hoisted up their tunics so as to be freer to run, and Leo smiled as he caught glimpses of their short trousers beneath, because what came to mind, wrapped in a delicious and erotic halo, was 'novice'. The boys sang and shrieked. Thomas leapt to his feet, grabbed his shirt and ran after them. Leo stubbed out his cigarette and asked the waiter for the bill.

The Nazarenes had already left the square and were weaving their way through the maze of narrow streets in the old town. Leo ran but could not catch up with them. He could hear the pitter-patter of their echoing footsteps, and the children shouting, and he caught glimpses of blue cloaks, but when he thought he had finally caught up with them he found his way ahead blocked by a tiny alley with steep steps. Women giggled in windows and gesticulated to him showing him which way to go, but he always ended up in a narrow little street full of laundry hanging

126

from one side to the other, as in the Spanish neighbour-
hoods of Naples. He could hear them nearby and when,
through the silence that suddenly engulfed him, he heard
a dull rumble, like a seething crowd gathering momentum, he stopped in his tracks. Then he walked on slowly.

He ended up in the square in front of the cathedral,
surrounded by thousands of people waving palm fronds
and olive branches. Some were haggling over the price of
a candle or a religious icon. It all had the atmosphere of
a festival, with the entire forecourt filled with children,
families, old men, and women dressed in traditional
costume. The steps up to the cathedral were covered with
bundles of olive branches and the main doors stood out
sharply like a huge black mouth against the pale stonework of the façade. He pushed his way through the crowd
and went into the cathedral. He felt a blast of hot air.
There was an enormous candleholder at the end of the
main aisle alight with large white candles decorated with
sacred symbols. All around the faithful had placed
smaller candles, thousands of small flames burning and
merging with one another. Nearby was Thomas. He was
trying to stand a candle upright, using the liquid wax
flowing from the main candleholder to fix it. Leo went
towards him and stood there beside him without saying a
word.

A penitential procession was underway inside the
cathedral. Hundreds of people being herded along
between two wooden barriers. They were moving slowly
forward singing and kneeling as they went. Leo saw that
the line turned back on itself like a zigzag. Halfway along
the nave it changed directions, passed the apse and then

headed in the opposite direction towards a chapel, by the entrance, where there was a statue of the Virgin Mary. When the people in the procession reached the holy statue, they lightly touched the Virgin Mary, then kneeled and mumbled something, before finally setting down their burning candles. Thomas told him it was the Virgen de la Macarena, and in a while she would be taken up by the procession and carried as far as Las Ramblas.

Then they went back to their hotel, climbed the stairs to their room and leaned over the balcony. People had gathered on both sides of the boulevard. Prayers were being relayed through loudspeakers. On a terrace to their left, ten yards away, the radio station was broadcasting the proceedings. People singing *saétas* came to the microphone. It was a contest of virtuosity, to see who could hold the note the longest. The people below clapped and shouted. The noise of the birds in the aviary was drowned. Black cloths had been put over it and the feathered inhabitants reduced to silence.

The radio announced that the Macarena procession was about to arrive. First of all Leo saw the band, then the *pasos*, the processional floats filled with flowers, advancing slowly ahead of the crowd, with a monotonous and rhythmic swaying motion. Below them were the Costaleros. Leo only noticed them when there was a sudden change. People rushed under the floats, while others, sweating and exhausted, made room for them. The sacred images of Christ on the cross, Christ set down, the patron saints and statues of the Virgin Mary all moved slowly on, separated by a good fifty yards. Each float was preceded by its own contingent of Nazarenes.

They were all wearing their hoods, all barefoot, holding burning candles dripping wax on to their gloved hands. People tried to touch the floats and take a flower. Children collected the melted wax and made small balls with it which they threw across the street. Mounted policemen protected the procession, which was almost trampled underfoot several times.

When the floats reached a point beneath the balcony where the radio station was broadcasting from, they stopped and everyone looked up as if they were expecting something. At that moment, as the crowd fell silent, the tenor started singing the *saéta*. After a while Leo went inside and lay back on the bed. He could still hear the songs and high notes of the tenors. He was dazed and weary. Beyond the curtains blowing in the breeze he could see Thomas's body leaning on the balcony. Every so often Thomas came back inside and excitedly described what was going on below. He poured himself a small glass of sherry, added ice and stirred it with his finger. The sun was setting and the sky was orange. Thomas's body was a dark, back-lit figure now. And Leo was sad. He had a kind of foreboding.

Next day they felt like leaving Barcelona. They had driven out towards Saragossa. Leo realised that he had almost run out of cash. He knew that the banks would stay closed now until the following Tuesday, so he had asked Thomas to pay the bill, not knowing that Thomas also had virtually no money. Thomas had told him lightheartedly, as if it were the most natural thing in the world: 'Oh Leo, I can't. I've only got a hundred francs left.' And he had merrily followed the hotel porter down the hotel steps.

On the road to Saragossa Leo had driven in silence. He was annoyed. Thomas was map-reading and giving him directions. Leo would do the exact opposite to what Thomas told him. If he suggested he turn left, Leo drove straight ahead with his foot hard on the accelerator. If Thomas told him to carry on straight ahead, Leo pulled over at the next crossroads with his indicator flashing, to turn left. So Thomas eventually put on the Walkman headphones, crumpled up the map and threw it violently on to the back seat. Leo had stopped, without any warning, to drink a beer. Thomas had not gone with him into the bar. Then when Leo was getting back into the car, Thomas got out and said he had to go to the toilet. When they reached Saragossa, after about a three-hour drive, they were ready to slaughter each other.

They tried a couple of hotels, then decided on the Grand. Leo was sure they would either take Italian currency or his credit card. Once up in their room, beneath the gilded Baroque ceiling, the arguing started. It was visceral and violent. Thomas was not speaking. He had gone straight into the bathroom, turned on the hot water tap, and started to undress. Leo started to taunt him from the other room. Thomas made light of it. Leo leaned on the bathroom door and taunted him some more. He could see that Thomas was starting to crack, and that encouraged him all the more. Thomas plunged into the bath. Then Leo violently pulled back the shower-curtain and hissed at him: 'If you had more money I'd love you a lot more.'

An hour later Thomas was still in the bathroom. Leo was lying on the bed, drinking. He was furious, an unrequited mess of hatred and remorse. He felt better than he had in the car, because he had found a few able words to ward off what was really making him so sad. To all intents and purposes he had accused Thomas of being a whore, of living off him, with not a shred of dignity. And this seemed quite plausible to him. He had said what he had really thought – if only for a split second – when he had settled the bill at the Hotel Montecarlo. But from the moment he had managed, not without difficulty, to dupe himself, he also knew that the deeper reason for his distress was the fact that he had seen that Thomas, the person he loved most in his life, was incapable of living on his own, incapable of standing on his own two feet. He saw him as someone weak, someone who needed another person to lean on. He saw him as a vacillating person, as someone who was perhaps still too young. A ray of sunlight and hey presto! – sitting in a chair with his shirt off, drinking and sleeping. All very easy. And who had to look after him? Leo, that's who. Always Leo there to pick up the pieces, pay the bill in the restaurant, pay for his books and his shoes and his bottles of rum. Leo, always Leo. The rage was welling up inside him. Thomas was still in the bathroom and Leo was still winding himself up over the petty, niggling little details of their relationship. Everything seemed to represent an assault on him. Thomas seemed more and more insignificant to him, a jerk like any other, not worthy of his love. Thomas's superficiality was cheapening him, killing him off. All of a sudden he leapt to his feet in anger and ran over to the bathroom door. He started knocking at it, calling out Thomas's name and daring him to come out. And when he did not hear any response, he became even ruder, telling him he wasn't worth fuck all, either as a man or as a musician. Leo was in the grip of a rage that was making him destroy the very image of his partner with a self-inflicting ferocity that knew no bounds. The more he continued to yell at the closed door, the more loathsome he felt. Yet the only thing that satisfied him was venting his wrath.

Thomas eventually emerged from the bathroom, drunk and angry, leapt at him, threw him to the floor, and went to lie on the bed. He could hear Leo groaning. He took the packet of tobacco and nonchalantly rolled himself a cigarette. Then he went over to Leo and stuck the cigarette firmly between his lips. He lit a match. He moved it close to Leo's face and said in a quiet but firm voice: 'I'll kill you, Leo. I swear right now I could set fire to you.' He held the burning match close to Leo's hair, Leo thrust his lips towards the flame. He was speechless, and drenched with tears. 'But the fact is, Leo, I'd want to die with you.'

Thomas moved away towards the window. He opened it. The darkening evening light echoed with the sharp boom of dozens and dozens of large drums being beaten in front of the cathedral.

The beat of the drums became obsessive and rhythmic, one beat, a second, a third and then the cadence. It had been going on since early afternoon. And it would go on until midnight when the church bells were finally released to fill the heavens with the joyful sound of the Resurrection. Leo summoned up his strength, got to his feet and went to the window. He stammered something, asked Thomas to forgive him, and tried to wipe his eyes by rubbing them on Thomas's shoulder. Thomas eventually gave in, took him by the hand and led him into the bathroom. He filled the tub, undressed him and helped him climb into the bath. He washed his face with the bath foam, and massaged the back of his neck and his feet. Then he turned off the light and got into the bath as well, squeezing in next to Leo, putting his arms round him, laying his face close to Leo's mouth, a little hesitantly, to give him a kiss.

At about eleven that night they went out, famished. They followed the rumble of the drums right to the square in the heart of the old town. They sat at a restaurant table and washed supper down with two litres of strong bloodred wine. Then they strolled through the city arm in arm, together again, united against the chill of the evening. Everywhere there was a feeling of festivity as the Resurrection fireworks exploded on to the sky above. They went back to the Grand Hotel and played bingo until the small hours, in the huge state room with its dozens of large round tables. They won and lost, all at once. They were like maniacs. They laughed because they did not manage to follow the cascade of numbers being called out. They repeated them out loud, checked their cards and the closed circuit screens which showed the draw. The people all round them, dressed in long gowns and dinner jackets, looked at them with distaste. Thomas and Leo went on drinking spirits, and then ordered a sweet and some wine. When the girl came round selling the bingo cards, they greeted her merrily and drove her crazy, because none of the cards was the one they wanted, none of them had the lucky number. At three in the morning a waiter helped them up to their room. They fell into a deep sleep until the following morning.

On Easter Day Thomas insisted that they go to the bullfight. 'Vamos a los taros' he shouted, leaping across Leo's body prostrate on the bed. Leo called the doorman and managed to buy two tickets. Thomas was overjoyed and yelled his head off all through the massacre. That evening there was not a restaurant in the city that was not offering braised bull or other slaughtered animals. In the end they went to one of those low dives that Leo loved, with wooden tables, wine by the jug, people coming and going, playing pinball machines, with men getting drunk as they mindlessly watched the TV. A woman emerged from the kitchen bearing two steaming bowls of dark and highly spiced meat, into which Thomas and Leo immediately dunked chunks of bread. The woman beamed at them. Every so often she drifted over to their table to urge them to eat more. She poured wine into their glasses, fetched more bread and brought them platefuls of salad. Thomas said it was all wonderful. At the end of the meal they discovered that the meat they had tucked into with such relish was the bull's testicles. Thomas started to laugh and joke. They left the cantina arm in arm and strolled through the alleys of the old town.

They came upon a group of very young pissed soldiers with their shirts open, buttoning up their trousers as they came spilling out of a brothel. The prostitutes were teasing them from the windows and tossing vegetables and scraps of paper into the street. Below the soldiers joined arms and sang. Thomas stopped, curious. Leo had to pull him forcefully away to the other side of the street.

They went back to the hotel, played bingo for a while and retired to bed. It had been a great day, but during the bull-fight Leo had once again seen the colours of his Barcelona dream. That particular red and that particularly deep, metallic black had appeared on the hollow flank of the bull. And the white foam flowing from the exhausted creature's jaws. He had seen the colours bloom on the animal's hide and spread over his entire field of vision until it filled it completely.

At the back of the bullring, after the corrida, he had watched the dead animals being drawn and quartered. With large hooks through their hocks the carcasses were hoisted on to pulleys and pushed along an overhead track amid the clanging of chains and metal. They were butchered with deft and powerful strokes from long knives, then skinned and bled. The large heads with their ears chopped off were tossed into a corner, the black eyes misted over and now veiled by a solid, whitish membrane. The tongues that hung from the clenched jaws were dripping with blood that flowed like a foaming, steaming cascade into the waste chutes. A few minutes after they had been dragged by the horses out of the bullring, these huge beasts were no more than shapeless chunks of flesh to be sold off to the city's butchers. There was still so much blood. And so much blackness.

Leo walks alone through the colonnades of his home town. He has to say hello to almost everyone he sees, because he knows them all, and they all know him. He does not stop. He gives a quick nod of the head to his father's friends and his mother's friends, to the occasional relative, to the brothers and sisters of his own friends, to the shop assistants who work in the stores in the middle of town, to the watchmaker and the bartender, to the pharmacist and to one of his former high-school teachers, to his old basketball coach, to the deputy mayor, to the librarian from the municipal library, to a bunch of young men who play in a rock group, to a woman who used to be one of his classmates, and to her mother trailing along a few yards behind her. And when he ventures into the part of town that he likes best, where the colonnade ends suddenly at the entrance to the Church of St Francis, even there he meets someone he knows. The antique dealer, the parents of a friend, someone he used to play mah-jongg with, a music teacher, someone who beat him at ping-pong twenty years ago, and someone who beat him at tennis fifteen years ago. This is why he is happiest walking around the town at night, when he knows there is only a slim chance he will bump into anyone he knows, apart from the odd friend in a bar or coming home from a party or a dance-hall. In these moments, in the stillness, with the overhanging lights of the streetlamps penetrating the darkness of the *corso* like great big illuminated umbrellas, with the sweeping arches of the colonnades, with the shiny marble stonework that makes them look like halls of mirrors, with the belfries and towers lit up by orange floodlights, his home town looks disturbingly like the set of a solemn Nativity play that he once saw and experienced with others.

The procession emerges from the church, preceded by the litanies being broadcast by loudspeaker along the way. He reaches the square and stands by a pillar as if

136

trying to hide. He feels awkward and perplexed. He sees the arrival of the parallel lines of choirboys, with their white surplices and their black robes, walking along beside the gigantic cross, fifteen or twenty feet long, being carried along on the backs of three men. The cross itself is black and a purple vestment hangs from the crosspiece.

Some nuns guide the children along the winding route of the procession. They slow the pace, cautioning the children with their glances to be quiet, and urging them to pray. There are not more than thirty children, who seem to be enjoying themselves. They proceed to the middle of the *corso* and smile at the onlookers. When Leo was part of those processions, he too used to start off from precisely this spot, at the head of the procession. But he does not recall any specific moment in particular. Only when he sees the statue of the Virgin Mary moving forward above the heads of the crowd, her heart pierced with daggers, does he feel a thrill. The sacred image stands out starkly against a forest of large poles bearing aloft the emblems of the Passion. Other slightly older choristers carry these banners, each one showing a different symbol: the nails, the crown of thorns, the sponge of vinegar, the dice, the lash, the white robe of the everlasting child . . . On one occasion it was he who carried one of these emblems in the procession. He remembers how an icy rain poured down. The mother of one of his friends had come running up to them from the back of the procession with an umbrella to protect them. But the prior had waved her abruptly away, blocking her path: 'They must learn to suffer!' And the woman had run off under the colonnades, and he and his friend, drenched from the rain and numb with cold, had walked on right to the entrance to the church.

He had also carried the Virgin Mary, when he was barely a teenager. It was a statue of Her hoisted up on to a massive wooden throne. Throughout the whole procession he had only been relieved once and the shoulder where the shaft rested ached. His arm was stiff and his legs were about to give way beneath him. With all his might he tried to stay upright, and he noticed that all the other boys were gritting their teeth too. Then, two hundred yards from the church, he finally saw a fellow chorister who was waiting to relieve him for the last leg, and he gritted his teeth just a bit harder, telling himself he only had just a couple more yards to go. He smiled because he was reliving it all. He almost shouted out loud as he watched the boys about to relieve the bearers coming closer, ready to change places. But at that moment the boy, a fair-haired fifteen-year-old, who was carrying both the shafts ahead of him, like an ox carrying a yoke, shook his flushed face and said: 'Go away, go away, I can do it on my own!' The others tried to persuade him otherwise but his mind was made up. He carried on shaking his head, almost doubled over by the strain, until the other chorister gave in and shooed away the relief teams. Right then he felt he might faint. He saw the chances of carrying his huge effort through to the end fading, and he glanced at his friend, and asked him what was going on. The other boy answered that they could do it on their own, right to the end. He asked him again and even a third time why they could not be relieved, but he knew from the start that it was a pointless question. He started to cry and kept on walking, stumbling a little. And he kept on saying to himself 'I'll never do it, I'll never do it', but what frightened him most was not the physical pain, which was acute and exhausting – he could feel the wooden shaft digging into his very flesh – but the shame of it. If he had given in, none of his friends would ever look him in the eye again. Once more he would have been the weakling, the cry-baby, the outcast. He would have no more friends. At school no one would talk to him and everybody would sneer and mock at him in basketball games and in church.

So he made an even greater effort because he had no other choice: he could not give up, and yet there was no way he could go on. In the church, when they finally relieved him of the weight of that effigy that he would then curse for years to come, Leo did not feel proud of having done what he had done, as did the others who were exhausted, too, but pleased with themselves for having lasted the whole course. Instead he felt deeply humiliated, really wounded deep inside himself, because he had been forced to put up with something that went against his whole nature, because he had been forced to show the others the most stupid and meaningless thing in the world – that he was just like them. Such an effort for something that for him was completely worthless. Now as he watches that macabre statue swaying along, supported by the boys beneath – today's fifteen-year-olds – he sees himself in a blaze of memory as a boy once more. And in the line of people he has joined he sees the different stages of his painful growing-up in the world. When he sees, far off, the black-draped catafalque with the prostrate statue of Christ Crucified, protected by a tall canopy held aloft by twelve men, he realises that he never reached this point of the procession. He stopped somewhere before this. He realises that life made him give up a little before he reached that part of the procession that has always been reserved for grown men.

The people around him kneel as the pall-covered coffin passes by, preceded by the priests and the canons. He stands still, stiff and tense. The band is playing a funeral march, slow and rhythmic. He looks at the statue of Christ and feels overcome by an agonising sense of piety, because his mind goes back to Barcelona, and Thomas's body, and he is quite sure that on that faraway day he was already attending the funeral of his partner. The recollection is a violent one, made all the more torturous by the band's funeral dirge. And there are no flowers, there are no festivities, just the harshness of a country tradition carried on without pomp or circumstance.

Inside the church, between two aisles packed with people and the smell of incense and candlewax, violins accompany the entrance of the catafalque. This particular piece of music is only ever played on this occasion. It has been that way for two hundred years, and he knows the music by heart. The orchestra solemnly starts playing, repeating the opening notes three, four times. Then the choir files in, ending with the tenor who starts singing the *Parasti Crucem*. The Reproaches follow on, one after the other, alternating between the chanting of the choir and the voices of the soloists. In one of them there is a passage for flute which thrills him much more than all the *Misereres* he has heard to date. It is a moment he would compare with the agony of mother Mary's silence at the foot of the cross. And it is something that makes him instinctively raise his eyes upward, and remember:

¿Quién me presta una escalera
para subir al madero
para quitarle los clavos
a Jesús el Nazareno?
(Who will lend me a ladder
to climb the cross
and remove the nails
from Jesus of Nazareth?)

The statue of Christ Crucified has been laid at the top of the chancel steps, at the foot of the high altar. Four men are standing at each corner of the catafalque. People are crowding on to the steps. At a precise point in the music the priests reach the statue, kneel down and kiss it, thus initiating the ritual that will conclude the Good Friday celebration. In a confusion of pushing and shoving, chatter and shouting, chanting and praying, signs of penance, genuflexions and bowing heads, the people make their way to the statue and kiss the wounds on Christ's feet and brow, body and hands.

Sitting on a pew in the side aisle, Leo watches the hundreds of people bending over that dead body and he recalls those times when, as a boy, he reached the top of the steps and bent over to kiss the face of Christ. There was a girl and he held her hand secretly in the thick of the crowd, knowing that no one could see them. Together they bent over to kiss the face of the statue, but it was not

141

until later, outside the church, beneath the lime trees lining the boulevard, that he had smelt the scent of a skin that was not like his, and the warmth of another body holding him close. She, need one add, was the most beautiful girl in the town, the tallest of them all, with the bluest eyes. And he had fallen in love with her in that awkward, guilty way that teenagers do. He did not desire her, because he was still not aware of the urges within his body, but he loved her in a strange and troubling way. He could not find things to say to her, he just wanted to hold and squeeze her hand. And it was the thing he liked most of all, to hold it tenderly and warmly – to slip his fingers into the pocket of her thick coat, as if it were some cosy nest, and there find his girlfriend's fingers already waiting to play with his, and interlock with his and tickle him lightly around the nails, and bunch her hand into a fist in his open palm. It was just knowing that there was someone in the world, on that walk along the *corso* or in the darkness of the cinema, who was waiting for him, someone who was fond of him. And someone who was protecting him.

But then, when he was young and inexperienced, when he lived in dread of growing up in the world of men and grown-ups, when he was no more than the sum of his 'own weaknesses', back then, when he fondled his young girlfriend, he was afraid of being found out, and he was ashamed of the feelings he harboured within himself. The older boys mocked and sneered at him, threatening to take his trousers down just to make sure that he was really a man, so improbable did it look if you judged from his still boyish look, with his smooth cheeks and hairless armpits. As a result he did not feel he deserved that girl. After a few months, in the summer, when she moved up from the secondary school to the high school, she had chosen another boyfriend, who happened to be Leo's best friend. But Leo did not give up hope. He went on being in love with her. The difference was that now he could be secretly in love with her, from the wings as it were. He could steal into her new relationship as a confidant to both her and her new boyfriend. That way he could become the vital link. So his best friend and his ex-girlfriend would both tell him what was going on between them. This position put him on both sides of the fence. When he heard both sides of the story from both parties, he felt strong because he had a precise role to play. Thus he thrived off the love affairs of others which would never be 'his affairs', but which, in a certain way, he was able to work out for those involved. By feeling at one remove, immersed in these problems and living with them, but always from a distance, like a separate beating heart, he found a way of observing and writing and, possibly, a way of growing up without being immediately put upon by the other boys.

On this hyperrealistic papier-mâché effigy, on this Christ Crucified, with the bleeding wounds, the crown of thorns, the holes of the nails, and the lacerated side of the body, was superimposed not only the image of Thomas in agony and dead, but also the image of another person whose funeral he is now attending, but now in silence. Because what his home town has carried through the streets in that procession and laid before the high altar is not the effigy of a divine body, but Leo's own dead body, the corpse of that boy who has never changed, a boy who has simply shed his skin, day by day, like plucking the petals off a flower. As a result he feels tense, and once more he experiences the one real feeling that he can have when he looks at the crowd: shame. He feels stripped bare, completely naked in front of the whole town. Everybody can see him, and the people go back to being the pharmacist, the schoolteacher, the house-painter, the antique dealer, the traffic warden. Everybody looks at him strangely, with suspicion and hostility. They insult him and snigger at him. As he faces them, once more, he is naked, blemished by pain and distress.

Christmas is just a promise. The mystery of the incarnation resides in Good Friday: the Passion, the oppression of the weak, the violence, the shame of being flesh and blood. Suddenly the awareness that he is attending his own funeral cortège makes him walk quickly away, back hunched, away from all those people who are realising what a hypocrite he is, what a paltry wretch. He feels humiliated and defeated. Without any hope of resurrection, either for himself or for Thomas. Nor, come to that, for that boy on the steps waiting to kiss Christ's face, who glowed with emotion as he squeezed the hand of his first real love.

On his thirty-first birthday – a bright, sunny September day that finds him in a seaside town on the Adriatic coast, where shadows lie long across the beach and the light is like the light in a studio set for a pop promo; the things that come into his field of vision include a pale strip of sand, a large beach umbrella, a beach-bed with a burgundy beach-towel draped over it, fluttering in the breeze, and the blue line of the sea, a deep blue that reminds him of the sky in the Dolomites – on his thirty-first birthday he has been alone for months, more than a year in fact.

When he was with Thomas he never asked himself about the deep-seated reasons why a person will live his life on his own, without having a family, without lovers. He does not have any children but, despite that, he can in no way be described as a person for whom something is missing. In the glorification of his present solitude, which he has been pursuing for months as something worthwhile rather than something required, he forces himself to investigate other forms of solitude in the hope that they might teach him how to behave. He wants to get the better of himself, but to do so, and in order not to find himself ever again swept away in the karma of falling in love – never again to utter those words that he had said to Thomas, 'I-love-you', to anybody else – he needs someone who will teach him, someone to square up to.

Come to think of it, he has always been alone, which is why he knows how to deal with it. He never has a problem knowing what to do with his time, or what to do at night. He likes sleeping, he enjoys writing and reading, and every so often he enjoys chatting to people he does not know. But he has never felt as alone as he has since he lost Thomas, because in losing Thomas he has lost something that made the long sequence of youthful solitude bearable. When he travelled across country to go to university he never really talked to anyone on those seemingly endless journeys. The same in class: he never dared to ask questions, or ask for something to be explained. And if someone turned to him to ask something as simple as the time of day, he would stammer a vague reply, as if he were in front of an exam board. Everyone seemed to be better than he, much better looking, much better off, and certainly much cleverer. He would laugh at their quips, follow them at a distance into cafés and pizzerias, and watch them. Nobody was aware of his presence and years later, when he happened to bump into one of those students somewhere in Italy, they would never recognise or remember him. He, on the other hand, would immediately recognise them, regardless of the changes wrought by age, children, marriage and a career, because in the act of recognition he would refer back not to idle chatter or the odd occasion, but to the idea he had formed of that person, the idea-of-himself that everyone carries around with him until the grave. At such moments he had the precise impression of having passed through his university years like a ghost, and this was the direct result of the way his personality had developed. In some ways he had managed to get by by remaining aloof, as he had in his boyish love affairs. The years of apprenticeship were important in this respect too. Because he did not achieve anything concrete, be it something accomplished, or some kind of a relationship. He did not realise that the suffering was enriching him and that he was developing in an inward direction as a person. He would rather have made love, had fun, and branched out into emotional experiences and political quests, but instead he ended up tense and repressed, working on the mystery of his own solitude and aloneness, unaware that in so doing he was getting closer to the most palpable seam of that other reality that we call art.

He did not spend time with anyone. He went to the cinema and lived in a rented room in the suburbs. Not having someone in his life certainly hurt him, someone to embrace and love, someone with whom to create a sense of sharing. But he did not feel lonely, because he still had that special strength that Thomas's death had now stolen from him. And when the time had finally come to have erotic dealings with other people, he had found himself strangely at ease, and natural, and moved by the very pleasure of it, as if he had always been involved in such acts. And then in the succession of letdowns and small-time, seasonal cruising, when he felt very low, looking for a partner and returning to his room alone, he once again felt that something was pulling him onward, and this stopped him losing his self-confidence altogether, as well as his trust in others. He carried on nurturing his aloof steadfastness because in both instances – in the years of apprenticeship as well as in the period immediately following his assumption of adult reality, what kept him going in both work and love was the thing that had enabled him never to feel truly alone: his imagination – and that was what he had now lost.

In this respect his solitude is different now to any other solitude he has ever experienced or achieved in his life. He is aware that his imagination is dead. He is conscious of having lost it. And he has lost it in the face of the death of his lover, in the face of the one and only thing that might have been able to sort out that long, decade-long problem, that innermost sclerosis of hopes and dreams alike – the fear of having to die, the fear of being already dead.

But here, by the sea, hidden away in an apartment surrounded by thousands of hotels with corny names, in a small town whose name Bella Marina smacks of cheap dreams, he feels calm, as if, in his aloofness, he were strolling along the shore of some paradise lost. He is looking for the crowds, the hubbub, the bright lights, and in particular disco music and people dancing until first light, bodies having fun, bumping together, trying to intertwine themselves, and at the same time he feels exactly as if he is in the middle of a desert. He feels absolutely no interest in what is happening before his very eyes. Or, put another way, nothing he sees affects him. He feels it all as part of his own solitude. Yet the show that unfolds by night, and the night-people themselves help to keep him from being depressed.

He knows that all around him, even if they are light years away from what he is experiencing, other people are carrying on with the rituals of their lives, they are wasting time, they are trying to enjoy themselves, they are trying to fall in love and be happy somehow. He does not mind all this. He is glad that there is still life to be lived for other people. Even if at about six one morning, walking along the shore among the first bathers clad in their tracksuits and the last lovers quietly heading back to their hotels, he feels the weight of his own years like some sort of revelation. It has something to do with the waves of the sea breaking on the shore and leaving seaweed and small dead fish behind. He feels sterile. He will not bequeath any children to the world. He will not watch a small person who looks like him growing up as the years pass, a person who bears his name, and who will fondly remember him as he looks at an old photograph.

One night, in the apartment next door, he hears the members of a family hugging and saying 'Guten Nacht' to each other. He saw the shadows of a mother and daughter cast against the other wall of the terrace. They were holding each other in a typically feminine way with their arms at their sides and their forearms raised perpendicular to their bodies, like people handing out clothes or material. Their hair mingled. Then the daughter kissed her father and again he heard the same words as clear as a bell. 'How often,' Leo thought, 'did your father and mother say goodnight to you like that? Never, because you were already at college at that age.'

So it is possible he has returned to these parts because they remind him of a 'summer camp'. Holidays without parents. Along the coast he sees the huge buildings beached like ocean-going liners in the scrap-yard. The windows are unshuttered, the walls are full of holes, and the paintwork is flaking from the salt air. Some of the buildings still have enclosures round a stretch of beach. The façades of others bear the names of iron and steel companies from the North or workers' associations or co-operatives. Still others are like a throwback to Fascist architecture. Towards Cattolica he sees a summer colony built in the form of a sail. It now houses a disco.

As he compares his life with the lives of others, in this period, he cannot shake off the image of a 'college' or 'camp', as if the acceptance of solitude entailed giving up not so much sex and love, but more the parental figures in his life, his mother, and his own illusion. When he hastily prepares a meal, only half concentrating, without laying the table, he is aware of the meanness of his own supper and that makes him feel hemmed in as if he were at college. When he receives a guest – a friend who boasts about his own independence – and when he watches him arranging his wash things and placing his own soap apart, and his aftershave lotion and his shampoo and his eau-de-Cologne, Leo thinks back to the boy in the holiday camp who, just to survive, was forever forced to christen his own things with a 'this is mine, and this is mine too'. In so doing he defended his things from other boys and claimed his own territory. Then he realises that for most people the conquest of independence is at the expense of generosity, as if the proud outcome of 'I can do what I like' ended up being solitary suppers with a plate of rice and bread rolls. Ended up – and this is the clearest image that Leo has – as toothpaste tubes that the college-boy squeezes desperately right to the very end.

The sense of ownership that he sees in other forms of solitude seems exaggerated to him. In some people it becomes nothing more nor less than stinginess. In others there is something essential about it. And in others still it becomes parsimoniousness or takes on the form of neurosis to do with tidiness, cleanliness and a maniacal attention to the arrangement of both things and feelings. It is as if solitude had constructed within the heart of the individual a whole atlas of road works, cul-de-sacs, one-way streets, dams and earthquake barriers, in such a way that any feeling or new object has a preordained route, so that it can move around without causing any damage.

One day a divorced friend with whom he was staying said to him: 'I needed to do things for myself. I think it's important to be able to get on with things on your own. Do things just for yourself.' And Leo had appreciated his choice because he thought that any total dedication to other people revealed a kind of perversion. Moral expressions like 'love of humanity' or 'loving other people' seemed meaningless to him, because for him it was impossible to love other people as some abstract entity. Leo wanted to love just one exclusive presence in the world, a presence that was certain, definitive and part of his history: Thomas. He wanted to love once and for all and, even if he did not fancy deluding himself, he felt quite capable of doing just that. The world was full of unpleasant people, enemies, loathsome people, boring people and evil people. And he had no intention whatsoever of loving any such people. Because he did not regard them as examples of his species, or his kind.

The words his friend had spoken had encouraged him. Leo also wanted to see to his own things, his own life. Then one morning, while his friend was still in the shower, Leo started to make coffee, heat the muffins and look for the sugar and honey among the pots and jars. He looked out of the window above the sink at the garden and he thought about typical American houses with their large kitchens and huge freezers and, in particular, windows like these, and in his own way he was happy with this rekindled keenness when he sensed behind him the presence of his friend in his bathrobe, an insidious presence like a watchman or an inspector. It was his host's upbringing that prevented him from saying out loud: 'Mind those china cups! Get the honey, it's there, down there. No, that's not the right heat for the toaster!' What the silent presence of his friend, rubbing his hair, told him was precisely all these things. And then, as if caught in the act of stealing some jam or biscuits from a cupboard at college he left the kitchen saying, with an embarrassed smile: 'You get breakfast. I must use the bathroom.'

Leo realises that his need for solitude cannot cut him off altogether from other people. He is trying to find an answer to the need he feels to be with himself. He wants to carry on being generous and available and open, even if he is aware that it is not easy to reconcile such different demands. The fact is that solitude is changing him. He says: 'You're thirty-something, Leo. Your body does not react to things like it used to. You don't have that constant desire to find things out any longer. You don't have that desire to explore, and see people and different places and different landscapes. Your thirtieth year is giving you a new maturity.' Leo resorts to such justifications when he realises that for months now he has not been eating in the dead of night, he no longer cooks at three in the morning, an engrossing silent time he has a soft spot for, with his ear still deafened by disco music, and his head humming, concentrating for endless minutes on something said at the bar, or on someone's smile. Leo is in fact aware that age is relative and that what is swaying him is not a biological process but the hardening, the settling of a pain that is always with him, a pain that blends with the ageing of his cells, a pain that is still reluctant to work itself out, and disappear . . .

One day Hermann comes to the sea on a visit. Leo has managed to track him down and has invited him to spend the weekend. When they talked on the telephone they did not say much to each other. They joked about the fact that they have not seen one another for years. They talked about mutual friends. And then in the end Leo said: 'I'd like you to come here, just for a few days. I've got a big apartment.'

Hermann said: 'Fine. I'd like to see you too.'

When they finally meet, they talk for hours, through the whole afternoon and then for most of the night. Leo discovers that having Hermann there is good for him. He feels like joking, going back over the moments they shared together, explaining things, talking about the moment they decided to split up – something Hermann still holds against Leo, with a calm that Leo would not have thought him capable of. They are like two soldiers returning from war. They have spent days on end courted by death, as if in a trench, seeing their comrades die or just disappear.

Their thoughts hark back with a mixture of nostalgia and tenderness to the dark days of their relationship. Just like two soldiers who meet again after many years and remember only their drinking sessions in the barracks and nothing whatsoever about going into battle. If someone were to say to them, 'But you might have died. Others ended up dead, you know,' the two of them would fall silent, bewildered and upset, and then all of a sudden burst into incredulous guffaws of laughter. They have survived and they can recall everything like a dream. Like something that has nothing to do with them any more. So when Leo mentions Rome, Hermann laughs and covers his face with his hands and shakes his head repeating: 'I can't believe it! Did I really do that?' They changed. They are different. Hermann is also grappling with being thirty.

Leo does not talk about Thomas. Every now and then their discussion brings him to the brink of remembering, and every so often he is on the verge of saying 'Thomas used to say, you know, that . . .' but he stops himself just in time and manages to change the subject. Late in the afternoon they go down to the beach.

They lie on beach-beds. Hermann's skin is very white and Leo looks at it as if he were looking at a familiar object, something he has known at a vital moment in his life and that he is now rediscovering after many years, still intact in its particular loveliness. They listen to a Sandie Shaw tape with earphones plugged into Leo's Walkman. Now and then their eyes meet, but swiftly turn away again. They both know that they will end up in bed together, either that night or the next day. They know they will not part again before they have tried to repeat the miracle of the attraction that kept them together for all those years. And the moment comes on the following day, in the hot, sensual stillness of early afternoon. They court each other as if for the first time. It is a little awkward, with neither of them daring to make a move. Leo suddenly feels his heart beat faster when Hermann sits down beside him on the bed. They take each other's hands and embrace.

When Hermann leaves, Leo says goodbye at the station knowing full well that he will not go looking for him, or rather he will not see him again for quite a while. In the three days they have spent together he has felt content for

154

the first time since Thomas died. For the first time since then he has made love and spent time with someone else. But he knows that his relationship with Hermann cannot go any further. They could try and live together again, because they are both in no doubt that they are fond of each other, and that they desire each other. But one day their lives went off in separate directions, and nothing can ever bring them back together again. Those days they spent close together, and at one with each other, in a way that never happened before, those days have for Leo marked the end of his relationship with Hermann. For he senses that he still loves Hermann, that he will love him for the rest of his life, but he knows that there would never be any hope with Hermann. He would always be late for meetings, he would always be missing trains, and forgetting things left, right and centre, and probably being unfaithful too. But most of all Hermann is still the embodiment of his old myth, of his fantasy, of the Vondel type, and he knows that all that died its own death with Thomas. In Vondel Park, these days, there is no longer anybody sitting on the ground playing a guitar or a flute. Nobody is noiselessly dancing behind the bushes, caught in the web of their psychedelic trip. There is nobody trying to sell you dope or necklaces, or trying to tout tickets for some concert. Today, if you cross Vondel Park, it even seems smaller. That same willow tree with its branches dipping into the water of the lake seems to be more isolated, as if they had cut down the beech and oak trees around it. Over on the far side there is a group of kids coming his way. They have armbands and white signs on their chests like athletes. They are holding nets and bamboo rods and wicker cages and a ladder. They belong to a group for the protection of birds in Amsterdam. They climb up the trees, check the nests and record how many eggs and broods there are. They make notes about the birds: they take the injured ones to the veterinary ambulance of their group; the ones that are poisoned by the polluted air are taken off to the country. The dead ones are thrown into the rubbish bins.

That same evening, alone again, before he drops off to sleep, Leo churns over the thought that has been haunting him for months now: 'And what if it were you, Leo, who had killed off your ideal, using Hermann and Thomas as the sacrificial lambs? Would they not be your innocent victims? And you, because you have not been sacrificed, and because you are the sadist who desperately murders those you love most, why do you want to be on your own?'

All this frightens Leo, and he has no answer to it for the time being.

The following year, after spending a winter in Milan trying to get a few projects off the ground, Leo accepts Michael's invitation to take a trip to the United States. Michael has left Paris. He has been living for a while in Washington D.C., playing in a club, and spending the weekends in a small wooden house by the ocean, in Delaware. When they meet again, Michael asks Leo discreetly about Thomas, and Leo is at a loss for an answer. Then Michael smiles and tries to sidestep the awkward moment by saying: 'It's okay. I understand. Thomas isn't with us any more.' And Leo nods, as if he is apologising: 'That's right, he isn't with us any more.'

One night, while they are having a meal with some of Michael's friends in one of the usual gay restaurants, his head throbbing with too many Martinis, he picks up on a reference to a place that is off the beaten track, some way away. He asks more about it and then pesters Michael to go along with him, that same night.

The others do not go with them. They say their good-byes outside the narrow entrance to the Blue Boy. Michael leads the way to the club. On the ground floor there is a disco with a small dance floor, TV screens showing video clips, a bar with a long counter, pinball machines and video games. On the floor above there is a piano bar. The lights are dim, and a few people are sitting round the wooden tables. To gain access to the next floor you need a ticket. Leo is curious. They walk down a passage with dim, reddish lights. At the far end there is a crush of people. Above their heads, swathed in clouds of smoke and the light of the spots, Leo glimpses the half-naked body of a dancer.

Michael orders a couple of beers and tries to push a way through the crowd. Leo follows him, his eyes glued to the young man dancing. They manage to make their way to the runway beneath which there are tables with silent men staring at the dancer, their heads turned at almost a hundred and eighty degrees. Against the walls of the room, which is some thirty feet long, there are stools and small round tables soaked in beer. Some people are leaving and Michael manages to secure two seats. Leo orders two more beers.

The dancer moves out along the runway, alternating acrobatic positions with ordinary dance movements. He

157

looks at the audience, smiles, meets the stare of a man and holds it while he gyrates his pelvis, then falls to the floor, gets up again, and makes his way back along the runway. In the middle of the room a sphere of mirrors turns lazily, sending beams of light over the onlookers and across the dancer's body. Now and then coloured spots flash on and light up the whole place.

With the first performance over, the lighting suddenly changes. The dance music has a slower beat, and the runway is dark. The boy moves snakelike along it, bending and flexing, arching his back and miming a sex act. He is wearing a coloured t-shirt and a pair of black cyclist's Bermuda shorts. On his legs he has a pair of very thick white woollen socks and basketball sneakers, the type with high ankles. More complicated, more insistent, more seductive are the movements he makes to take his Bermudas off. He is a muscular, fair-haired young boy with a crew-cut and not a hair on his smooth chest and legs. He cannot be more than twenty. There is something inviting about his handsome face. He stands in the middle of the runway and slips out of his trousers doing a kind of belly dance, letting the spotlight fall first on the pale whiteness of one buttock, then the other, and then his genitals. When his shorts finally fall down his legs, lodging over his calves, all that remains is a tiny black leather jockstrap. He dances a little more, playing with the strap and moving with dainty steps like a geisha. All of a sudden he vanishes behind the curtains. The music changes again and the spot shines down on the front of the stage. The audience, mostly men between thirty and fifty, light cigarettes and start talking. After what seems like a long minute the same young boy dashes out from behind the curtain and everyone claps and shouts and whistles. He wears only shoes and leg warmers. He has an erection and masturbates as he dances. Dollar bills are thrown from the tables close to the runway. He bends down, revealing his cock, practically touching the onlookers' faces with it. Or he flexes his legs and shows off his thighs. People in the audience can touch him. He lets them touch him for a few seconds, then takes their dollars and slips them into his leg warmers with a thank-you. Then he lies with his stomach on the floor and pretends to fuck, or he lifts his legs and moves his buttocks as if someone was penetrating him. He looks at his audience, blows kisses and beams smiles at them, and pockets their dollars. Then he exits and lets another young dancer take the limelight.

Michael asks Leo if he is enjoying the show. Leo says he is. He lights a cigarette. He does not feel like talking. The boy on stage now is black, quite tall, with the same kind of well-built athletic body. He is wearing a pair of jeans that are torn across the ass, a black leather jacket and a red band around his forehead. His hair is long and loose. He has the face of a model. While he starts to dance, the first boy, wearing no more than his G-string, starts to wander among the tables. He plants himself in front of a spectator, pirouettes a couple of times, shows him his cock, and rubs against his legs or sits on his knee. He refuses to move until the spectator gets out a dollar or two and slips them inside his jockstrap. When Leo sees him coming towards him his first instinct is to hide. He glances at Michael, because he is not sure what to do. He feels everyone's eyes on him, which gives him a sense of paralysis. The boy stares at him smiling, fondles his own nipples, hardening them, moves his tongue, spins and flexes, like a statue. Michael chuckles but Leo is rooted to the spot. He is thinking to himself: if I give him a couple of bucks he'll move on. But he does not want to put his hand in his pocket and pull out the bundle of bills and check to make sure he is not peeling off a fifty or a twenty instead of the expected one dollar bill. So he does nothing. He just hopes that the dancer will move on to someone else. And he does. Leo feels a whole lot better and downs another Budweiser.

But he does not feel at ease. An excited feeling of curiosity makes his throat feel tight. He feels poised, about to do something forbidden. As if he has to get past a No Entry sign. Instead of conjuring up images of entertainment, drunkenness, dancing, the word 'strip-tease' troubles him, as if it were something altogether sordid. Dirty and clandestine. He realises that it is a sensation that has to do with his childhood, way back in the fifties, when the word was uttered with caution and shame. There was a place in his home town called the Chez Vous. The police had shut it down, arresting the owner, the strippers, and customers from Milan, Bologna and Florence. His mother and father had never mentioned it but he knew about it, not least because a good-time well-off uncle of his had been involved. One day he had found a photograph with his parents in evening dress dancing in the midst of streamers and confetti. They were smiling at the photographer's flash. And his mother was very beautiful, her shoulders bare with a large satin wrap like a stole around her décolleté.

He had asked his mother what party the photo was taken at, and she had told him it was New Year's Eve at the Chez Vous. When she told him that he had felt deeply troubled because he could not believe that his parents had actually gone into that forbidden pleasure-dome, not even once. Like all children he lacked a temporal perspective, and he had superimposed two things – the strip shows and the New Year's Eve party – which had nothing whatsoever in common except that they had both taken place in the same nightclub, albeit years apart. So the innocent New Year party turned into the mythical forbidden *dolce vita* event of his home town.

He carries on smoking and drinking, but still does not manage to calm the swirling movement in his eyes as he stares at the body of another dancer. After the fifth boy has done his turn Michael decides to quit. Leo says good-bye to him. He stays on another hour, sitting on a stool, watching three more boys do their strip act, followed by a number where two more give an acrobatic display showing different lovemaking positions. Leo leaves around one a.m. The next night he again heads for the Blue Boy. He stops off in a bar for a gin and tonic, just to delay his excitement. Just to tell himself: 'They'll have started over there already and I'm happy to be right here.'

It is a Friday night and there has been a change of boys, as there is every week. They do the rounds of the clubs in the United States and Canada. They range in age from twenty to twenty-five. They come in all shapes and sizes and colours: black, mixed-race, Puerto Rican and white. Their physique is built in gyms: muscular legs, pronounced pectorals, well rounded biceps, supple

161

backs. The only thing that varies is the structure of their bodies: some are taller than others, some are long-legged, others thickset and powerful like bulls. Then there is the vigorous Californian surfer type, the moustachio'd working-class type, the farmer type with a red kerchief knotted at the neck, and the fashion-conscious model type with his English-style haircut and op-art jockstrap. Every night Leo is in the middle of them all, perched on his customary stool, every night, handing out dollars, rubbing up against their bodies, smiling and knocking back beers. After three nights they know who he is. When the time comes to circulate among the tables the boys say hello to him and wink as if to say: It'll be your turn soon. When they strip on the runway, they see him among the audience and try to catch his eye. When they do they stare hard and do a few phallic acrobatics as if just for him. Leo gets rid of dollars, one after the other. Then it all happens over again: the boy arrives, rubs up against him, strokes his cheek, turns and says: How you doin' handsome?, and then shows him his ass and everything else. Even the boys he does not fancy – because he has his favourites and those who do absolutely nothing for him – even when the little short one comes over to him, Leo gets over his awkwardness and slips some money into his pants, with the result that the little short guy keeps coming back for more. Leo has an absolute favourite: a long-legged, dark-skinned boy, probably from Puerto Rico. Leo finds his eyes quite beautiful and the shape of his lips perfect, generous and sensual. He is less muscle-bound than the others but he is the only one whose legs are covered with dark, curly

162

hair which highlights the contours of his muscles. In fact the thing he likes doing best, when the boy comes up to his table all smiles, is to spend a good long while caressing his thighs and his knees.

He drinks beer after beer and every so often has to go off to the washroom to relieve himself. When he returns to the now empty room – the boys are forever shortening the time their acts take to squeeze the last bucks from their audience – he finds himself face to face across the runway with a young man whom he noticed for days, always in an identical position. But he only really catches his eye now at this moment. He is drunk, sunk in his chair, with a whole bunch of dripping wet dollars under his beer glass. He is wearing a jacket, tie and waistcoat and has an overcoat draped over the seat. His hair is thin but long, with a sweat-matted lock over his eyes. He has a fat ring on his finger. He has a permanent smile on his face, as if frozen in a half-witted expression. The boys must know him pretty well by now because they treat him the way nurses treat an elderly chronic patient. They know he likes being touched between the legs, but not for too long. They all touch him there, mechanically, with a kind of polite offhandedness that amazes Leo. The man, who must be about thirty-five, keeps on smiling, drinking beer and slipping dollars into jockstraps. Leo is tired. His eyes are glazed and softened with alcohol. He looks up at the ceiling, takes the back of his neck in his hands and has a good stretch. It is precisely at that moment that it happens.

The ceiling is covered with mirrors. He has not realised this until just now. So he sees himself, pale as a sheet, in the midst of a desolate space full of empty tables, stools and bottles of beer. In that image he sees the drunk man with a naked boy on his knees. Mirroring himself in that double of himself and identifying himself with the young man, drunk and contorted, who is still smiling as if he were holding a puppet or a doll in his arms, he says to himself with a mixture of resignation and excitement: 'Okay Leo. Right here and now you too have started a career as an honest whore.'

The club is closing. The dancers, no longer naked but now wearing soft tracksuits or sports jackets, walk round the tables, drinking beer and chatting with the few remaining customers. One of the dancers is sitting right beside Leo. He is tall and well built with a massive neck. He is wearing black leather boots with studs on the heels. His head is completely shaven. He has on a pair of black leather breeches which show his buttocks and his genitals. His right wrist sports a black bracelet covered with chrome studs. All evening long Leo has watched him seducing and soliciting athletic men. He knows he has a cockring tight around his balls. But Leo had not noticed a small ring attached to his left nipple. The guy touches it lightly with a finger, making it swing and then gives Leo a cold, hard look and stretches out a hand towards his chest.

Leo feels confused because no leather type has ever looked twice at him. Leo does not like this kind of scenario much, either. But he feels excited because it is as if the guy recognises in him, in his bourgeois clothes, in his face, and in his eyes something that Leo is apparently not aware of. This is why Leo follows the guy out of the room.

Backstage there is a very narrow, steep stairway leading to the floor above where there is a fairly wide passage with mirrors on the walls, coat racks and metal seats. On the seats there are piles of clothes, holdalls and shoes. A dancer is slipping into a pair of jeans. A little further on in the shadows Leo recognises the Puerto Rican. He is sitting down, bent over, his long socks pulled down to the floor. Like a street kid he is counting his dollars: dozens and dozens of crumpled, creased bills like so many toffee wrappers.

They go into quite a large room where the far wall is divided up into three black plastic booths. One of them is open, with a black leather single bed, and a towel laid over it. The curtains to the other booths are pulled to and below them Leo gets a vivid glimpse of a man's naked legs. He hears groaning and moaning, and barely stifled cries. He does not know whether of pleasure or pain.

The dancer pushes him down on to the bed and yanks the curtain shut behind him. First he opens Leo's jacket, loosens the knot of his tie, unbuttons his shirt, and pulls his trousers halfway down his thighs. He keeps all his clothes on. It is as if he had just opened Leo up at the centre with a can-opener. Leo squeezes the man's arm hard. He pulls at his wrist with both hands, as if he were rowing a boat, and looks up. He feels cold. There is a white light on the ceiling. He feels a violent pain in his balls but the man swiftly covers his mouth with a hand, like a slap, stopping him from crying out loud. The pain shoots through him again, sharper and longer, and Leo starts to feel frightened. The guy slips a black condom on to him and starts to suck him. Leo shuts his eyes. That white light flashes on again. Fear and cold. They were moving him from a stretcher to the operating table. The pre-anaesthetic had not taken and he was terrified by the operation. A nurse had asked him if he wore false teeth and he had shaken his head and realised that his turn was about to come. They had pushed him into the operating theatre. The nurse had moved the stretcher close to the table and asked the staff already there to give her a hand. They all had their faces covered with small masks and in his dazed state he could hear them talking among themselves as if he were already dead. He looked at the huge light in the middle of the theatre and its round bulbs and he felt cold. He was freezing cold. Then a nurse had brusquely removed the sheet that had been covering him and he realised he was completely naked. They settled him down on the hard operating table and folded his arms across his body. He could feel them tying him down. The nurse was giving orders to a very young girl who seemed if anything more terrified than Leo. She was having trouble getting his wrist into the strap and the nurse snapped at her to get a move on with what she had been taught to do, and stop day-dreaming. Leo saw the girl's eyes and could see how afraid she was of being in this place. He could see at least six people wandering around the theatre, walking to and fro, glancing at the naked body waiting to be butchered, and then turning away. Never before had he ever had such a direct and blinding experience of himself as a corpse, as something anatomical. He reddened and felt himself sweating. The girl finally squeezed his arm and managed to insert the needle. The nurse told her she had done a good job: 'You mustn't be afraid. It's quite easy!' she said, encouraging her. But nobody asked Leo anything. He felt split in two, in a state of absentia. Before the girl moved away she took a small green cloth and tossed it over Leo's sex to cover it. He closed his eyes and breathed deeply, as if to thank her.

The man is tying something around Leo's prick. All Leo can feel is pain, acute, sharp pain. But he can also feel a strange tension, all focused there between his legs. His breathing is coming faster, as if from that place where all the pain is concentrated; and then it spreads out right through his whole body. His hand starts stroking the guy's shaven head. He gets to his feet and comes close to Leo. He is still wearing his black open breeches, and now his cock sticks out, completely uncovered. Leo grips it, squeezes it, and the guy lets out a deep, short sigh, like a low bellow. Leo sees him now standing close beside him; he looks at his powerful chest and a rivulet of sweat running from his pectorals down to his navel. His strong, massive neck is swollen with veins. He watches the studded hand that is slowly masturbating him. He feels close to orgasm, but it is as if he were repeatedly reaching the moment of no-return without ever ejaculating. The pain grows stronger and sharper, but he wants more, and more. He begs the guy to give him more. The guy grabs one of Leo's nipples and starts to squeeze it; then he pulls it and bites it. He tightens a neckband around Leo's throat and pulls it slowly. Leo is afraid he might choke. He suddenly feels his head exploding, swelling up with boiling hot blood. He is sweating. His eyes only see dimly what is going on and his breathing makes a dull gasping sound.

When it was time to fit the tubes into him, in the icy operating theatre, he was still conscious. He was alive in a dead body. A prisoner. He could not speak, he could not move his hands, but, as if in a dream, he could distinctly feel them bending his legs and talking across his body. Then he had felt as if something were suffocating him. He had tried to vomit, but something was tightening more and more and stopping him from breathing. And then, in those last rays of consciousness he thought: 'I'm choking to death', and he let himself drift off, but he still was not dying and that thing in his throat was growing larger until it was enormous and spreading, squeezing every part of him, and it seemed like a hundred years that he had not breathed a breath. He was in pain. Then, in a moment of calm, he had thought: 'It's not so hard, dying. It's all a dream.'

Now, too, on the single bed in that kind of clinic of perversion he felt the same sensation of limits, beyond which all that happens, God willing, is a loss of consciousness. He feels his cock erect and hard and strong, full of blood ready to spurt out, but feeling blocked. Everywhere in his body, even his blood cells, there is a feeling of discomfort that he does not want to give up, as if, finally, all the years of pain he has been through, ever since Thomas died, ever since he, Leo, was born, all that pain was becoming tangible on that narrow little bed, in that tense body, in his balls and in his throat, from a scrap of leather. He is incapable of going forward or back. He is blocked there, suspended between life and death, between

168

the pleasure of the expert touch of an honest torturer and the pain of a body that, unlike his brain, still does not know its own breaking point. Again Leo grips the man between the legs, squeezing his balls and slipping a hand down over his thighs. He feels like hitting him, hurting him. He starts beating on his body and the other man responds by squeezing harder and harder. The veins in his neck swell, his jaws are clenched, his eyes harden, and with sudden violence he says something in slang that Leo does not understand. Then he sees him take a small red phial, unscrew the top and inhale deeply from it, twice. Leo recognises the smell of poppers. He tries to resist and say no. He turns away but the task-master presses the bottle against his nostrils. Leo makes an abrupt movement and a few drops spill into his nose. He feels a strong burning sensation and a trickle of fire seems to find its way down his throat. The other man has turned purple. He is sweating, his head drenched and glistening. Leo waits for the effect to hit, which it does all of a sudden in a flash. And in that moment, with his chest virtually exploding with pain, the man without warning undoes the straps, lets go of his throat and Leo explodes in a violent soaring jet like a white arc merging with the ceiling. And he feels himself sinking, and sinking, a strange kind of sliding that is very fast and intense but also – as he suddenly begins to realise – comforting, as if his whole brain were coming proudly down from the highest peaks to the hush of a familiar valley. He is panting like a runner after a long race. He cannot speak. He bursts out crying, a mixture of sobs and tears and coughing, and when his frail voice tells the man that everything is fine he stammers the words with a voice he never thought he could have had: the voice of boy-Leo. A shrill, high-pitched, effeminate voice, a whimper buried deep in his pain, a whimper that his pain has brought to life again.

Leo stays three weeks in New York, in a small apartment on Fifth Avenue at 92nd Street. In the mornings he walks in Central Park or hires a bicycle and challenges passing cyclists to a race. In the afternoons he sleeps, reads and studies. And in the evenings he treats himself to a little European worldliness, meeting Italian journalists, or a group of professors of literature at Columbia University. Later on, at night, he goes down to the Village or St Mark's Place, and drinks a good number of beers in the bars. He watches videos or shows put on by small groups of transvestites. He does not talk to anyone apart from bartenders who like his Italian accent, which, for them at least, makes him still uncorrupted or sane. He organises meetings in his own head, spends an hour or more imagining how a particular person's life might be, the sort of things he must be fond of, what job he might have, and what kind of sex he likes best. But it is all trivial and the strongest sensation he has is the feeling that he should have stayed in New York when he was twenty, full of energy, with the desire to get up and go, and a constitution to match.

He decides to return to Milan. He has a sense of foreboding a few hours before he leaves New York. An image that irritates and troubles him. That same morning he had thrown a pair of old black winter boots into the garbage bin. He had bought them in Paris. He threw them away simply because he wanted to get rid of all excess baggage, and that pair of boots had been the first thing to go. He had not given it a second thought until the doorman called to tell him there was a taxi waiting for him, and he was checking to make sure the gas and water were off. He had squinted through the window, and there, down in the backyard, he had seen the garbage men tip the bags into a large bin. And it was then that he had seen his boots tumble into all that garbage, lying on the top for a moment before being buried by more refuse and carted off.

He was not at ease when he reached the airport terminal.

He was anticipating a full plane, and his fears were confirmed at the check-in desk. He was too late for a seat near an exit with some leg-room. While he waited he saw a group of about thirty girls and hoped they would not be on the same flight. He also saw a party of Tuscans and again hoped that they were flying with another airline. An hour later they all found themselves on the same airport bus.

While Leo was putting his hand luggage away a very tall man with thinning white hair and rosy, freckled skin, took the seat immediately in front. Definitely a handsome man, he was wearing a dark-blue double-breasted suit, and had a very soigné look about him – he had a large gold ring on his little finger, a pearl-coloured silk tie and a Rolex that must have been at least thirty years old. Soon after take-off, he rather abruptly pushed his seat back. Leo, who had a problem in planes because of his height, swore when the seat hit his knees. He called the stewardess and asked her to ask the passenger not to let his seat back quite so far, because he had nowhere to put his legs. The stewardess talked with the man, who apologised to Leo, and then asked him how tall he was. Leo answered pleasantly enough. He looked him straight in the eye. He thought he could not be more than sixty.

They chatted for a few minutes, Leo the more cautious of the two, for the man seemed to need to exchange a few words with someone else. The pretext for their exchange was their respective height, the inconvenience of being tall, and the problems posed by finding a long enough bed in hotels, and, even more so, a seat with enough leg-room on planes. But Leo was aware that there was more to their banter than this. And from one second to the next he waited for that something to reveal itself. It happened after a few minutes had gone by, while Leo sipped at what was to be the first in a long succession of gin-and-tonics.

Even though their conversation had not hinted at anything quite so brutal and extraordinary, what the man said was: 'I've got my son with me, in the hold.' And with the forefinger of his clenched right hand he pointed at the floor. Leo felt himself on the verge of fainting because he understood at once. In fact he found himself saying to himself: 'Okay. That's what it's about.' 'I've got my son's dead body in the hold,' the old man went on, staring desperately at Leo. 'I came to America to fetch him.'

The muffled hum of the engines came into the cabin like an oppressive drone. The man was weeping and wiping his tears with a white handkerchief. Leo was speechless. All he could do was mutter every so often: 'It's terrible. I can't believe it.' But the man did not hear him. He went on telling him about his son and how he had had to spend the last month at his dying son's bedside. He told Leo that his son was a government employee, that he was fifty, and that cancer had killed him in just three months. Leo's legs felt weak. He kept calling the steward, ordering gin-and-tonics, and smoking cigarettes. He hoped he would soon feel drunk, and be able to lie back in his seat exhausted enough to fall asleep, but nothing worked. The man was sobbing, in a way that was thoroughly proper and seemly, and Leo felt like bursting into tears too. The idea that beneath his feet, 40,000 feet up in the sky, there was a coffin with a corpse in it terrified him. He felt close to breaking point, but he knew that he could never quite let himself do it: the aircraft would not alter its route, they would not let him disembark, they would not settle him down, full of tranquillisers; in a first-class reclining seat. So he gritted his teeth hoping that the old man would collapse first. But the old man was a retired general. He was in his eighties and quite capable of staying the course. He said: 'Are you married? If you are, don't ever have any children. You'll never know what this pain feels like. You'd be giving life to something that would come to nothing. I don't believe in God, but I swear I'd have made a pact with him: my wife and I in exchange for the life of this son of ours.'

Leo kept silent, preferring to let the old man ramble on.

Every now and then they had to pull back from the aisle into their seats because the schoolgirls were running up and down. The group of Tuscans, at the rear of the plane, were singing and laughing. They were opening bottles of sparkling wine. The two of them turned their heads instinctively towards the sound of the pops, and then carried on talking.

'I'm eighty-two and I've never smoked a cigarette in my whole life. I've never drunk alcohol and I've always led a healthy life, even though I've served all over Europe, in the United States and in Brazil. I've played tennis all my life and I still keep active. And what's it all been for? Just so that one day I can carry my son below me here on this plane. That's all it's been for.'

Leo touched his arm but did not look him in the eye. He felt responsible for those eyes, glazed and red and filled with tears and horror. Leo thought of Thomas's father, and of Thomas, too, of course. When at last the old man, so athletic and healthy, sat down exhausted with his eyes buried in his handkerchief, Leo had a chance to go to wash his face and shed a tear. He went on drinking, he tried to eat something, he ordered a couple of cans of beer, and finally he felt a little better. He closed his eyes, but could not find sleep. They were showing the movie and the cabin was dark. But in front of him he could still see the back of the old man's head, with his white hair and pink freckles. He felt like stroking that head, he wanted to say something to comfort him. But he was angry inside. The man who had never smoked or drank had kept himself in shape just to bury his own son. What was unnatural about it all was

174

not so much the premature death of the younger man, but rather the forced survival of the older. And then he thought that he, too, had in a way buried Thomas. And that both he and the old man were murderers who, in some way or another, had controlled right to the very end the life of the person they most loved. Right to the moment when the body they had created was laid in the grave.

Then Leo feels that this sado-masochistic instinct is not a strange impulse, but possibly the purest and the sincerest perversion he has ever experienced. Because he is a torturer and he is the victim designate of that persecutor who bears his very own name. Hermann, Thomas, and anybody else, they are just the instruments of a torture that he has been inflicting on himself ever since he achieved a state of self-awareness: the instruments, in other words, of his own need to humble himself and die. His demand for happiness and love has killed other people: he has been unable to contain or divert this demand, or juggle with it with any skill. It is not just love that has died with Thomas, but his own personal strategy of love. All that lies ahead of him now is a career as a virtuous lecher. The satisfaction of specific needs that only alien people can procure for him.

In the darkness of the slumbering cabin, two sleepless, grieving figures are lit up by the small overhead lights. Two men whose pain is an absurdity that cannot be contained by words: in fact the very expressions that could be used to describe it appear to make no sense. An 'orphaned father' and a 'widowed lover' are travelling in that plane destined for Europe, though, of course, the destined plane may never fulfil its 'destiny'. Because both the old man and the young man are on a journey, with their corpses beneath their feet, heading towards that icy land where life appears to be nothing other than the void left behind by a paradise decayed and lost for ever.

THIRD MOVEMENT

Separate Rooms

After a two-year graduate course at the Paris
Conservatoire, Thomas had gone back to his family in
Munich. He was twenty-three and he was at a very delicate moment in his life. Much of his future would be
bound up with the decisions and choices he made in those
summer and autumn months. He had to decide on a city
to live in – whether to carry on in Paris, go back to
Munich, or give Italy a try. He had to decide whether to
accept a three-month tour in the United States, or whether
to carry on making classical music recordings in Berlin,
which were well-paid but thoroughly anonymous. Or
alternatively whether to have a go at a teaching career in
a music school, whether to apply for a job with a theatre
orchestra, or whether to start as a soloist, doing the
rounds of small provincial theatres, concert halls and
musical benefits here, there and everywhere in Europe.

Thomas's head was in a muddle. He tried to get Leo to
help him, but whenever he talked about it to him he just

got the usual 'Do whatever you feel is best', uttered in an irritable and bored tone of voice. It annoyed Thomas when that happened and they usually had a quarrel. In fact Leo found the whole situation painful precisely because he was aware that he could not solve Thomas's problems for him. That was why he preferred not to discuss the matter, even if that gave Thomas the impression that Leo was not interested in his life. Their relationship had been working okay now for two years. But for different reasons they were both heading off in new directions: Leo towards an inner, quiet awareness of the fact that he was thirty years old, and Thomas for the fullness of youth.

Leo was also aware that if Thomas was gifted, this would have shown itself: in an orchestra just as much as in a recording studio or among the students in a musical academy. So he kept his distance from a situation that he found upsetting, resorting to a certain level of Mediterranean fatalism. He tended to carry on just as if nothing were any different. He handled their rows by simply not taking part in them. In so doing, he was unwittingly preparing himself for the toughest and most difficult row his relationship with Thomas had to endure.

When they saw each other again in Milan, in early September, Leo was in pretty good shape. Tanned, slimmer, his muscles tighter, his liver in good shape. Thomas, on the other hand, was showing slight, even if almost imperceptible, wear and tear. The skin on his cheeks looked more taut than usual, and his eyes were yellowish and glazed. He had spent the summer dealing with his move from Paris to Munich, plus a few weeks in the mountains with his parents and a recording job in Bath. Leo and he had not seen each other for about seven weeks. What was more, Leo had not left Thomas the address of the house on a Greek island where he had spent the summer with Rodolfo and other friends. He had done no more than send a postcard to Munich. When they met up again Leo immediately felt guilty because he realised that, for too long, he had not thought of Thomas with his usual faithfulness and devotedness. He still loved him. He took him for granted, though, like a certainty in his life. But he could see that, perhaps even more than in the early days, Thomas needed some confirmation that they still had a relationship and that it was still alive. Without any such daily reassurance of his love, and without his persistent professions of affection, Thomas was like a plant without water: he faded and drooped.

There was deep melancholy that Sunday evening as the Munich train was announced. Leo hated goodbyes because he knew he could never define them and limit them to a contingency. Every goodbye became the reflection of other partings and other separations, from his mother, from his home, from the routine of certain periods of his life. He had to go with Thomas to the station. He could not face watching him leave the apartment with a taxi waiting outside. He wanted to go with Thomas as far as the door, touch him lightly one last time and help him on his way from the place to which they would both return as two separate and totally unknowable people.

There was a crowd of soldiers on the platform, on their way to the Veneto and Friuli. Holdalls and suitcases and rucksacks, arms tight round fiancées' waists or squeezing

179

hands, groups of friends passing round a bottle of grappa, or knocking back dozens of cans of beer, mothers, relatives, a few old ladies saying goodbye through the train windows as if their boys were leaving for the front. There were platoons of Alpine troops going back to barracks in Balzano, talking in worried voices about a special camp they had to go to in a few days' time. There was a group of young men all with the same squat physique, heads close-cropped, wearing jeans and sneakers. They were talking in Neapolitan dialect, running along beside the train and yelling out when they found an empty compartment. The train was already packed.

Students gazed with melancholy faces from the windows, at the fate that awaited them once their studies were over. They pored over books, as if trying to shrug off a nightmare. Girls, young company secretaries, nice respectable young ladies with knee-length skirts and light cardigans wrapped around their shoulders against the first chill, leafing quickly through women's magazines and trying to do a crossword. They seemed like hostages on that all-male train. They curled up into their seats and only looked up now and then with cross faces because someone had bumped into them.

Leo and Thomas made their way along the packed corridors looking for the carriages going to Munich. They finally found an empty seat and Leo helped Thomas put away his luggage. He held out his hand, kissed him on both cheeks and got off the train. Then he walked away without even waiting for the train to pull out of the station.

As soon as he was back home again he poured himself a stiff drink, put on the stereo and stretched out on the sofa. He tried to relax, but he felt strange, relieved of the weight of Thomas living with him, happy to be alone, and yet feeling a great emptiness, a sign of a loss. It was just then that he thought he heard a ring on the housephone. He got to his feet, turned down the music and waited. The bell rang again. And then he was sure it had something to do with Thomas. He saw him emerge from the lift, looking dejected and awkward, but at the same time with a lively, proud look in his eye. Thomas threw himself into Leo's arms and said: 'I want to stay here and live with you.'

Leo was surprised and speechless. He stroked Thomas's head idly, took his luggage and went in with him. Thomas was radiant. He walked round the apartment as if he were seeing it for the first time. In his own scheme of things, it was to be his new home. He would never again visit it like a guest. He would live in it. Leo could hear a trace of loathing in his voice as he asked Thomas: 'So you've decided to live in Italy?'

Thomas did not pick up on it, or at least he pretended not to. He wanted to live in Leo's country, close to Leo. He had made up his mind: this was his chance.

Leo went on pouring himself something to drink and said hardly a word. When night came, and the alcohol had softened him up, he kissed Thomas and thanked him for having decided to live with him. Next morning, along with feeling dazed and having a headache, Leo knew with painful brutality that he would never be able to live with Thomas in the same apartment. For the two years they had already spent together the geographical precariousness of their relationship combined with the fact that they lived apart had been a spur to staying together. Now he had to give serious thought to the notion of living together with another man. But he had no models to follow, no experience to recycle and fall back on in this stage of their relationship. He knew that the love he still felt for Thomas would not be enough on its own. They would tear each other to pieces and that was the last thing he wanted. They would hurt each other, and then they would leave each other high and dry. Living together meant believing in values that neither of them was capable of recognising. How would their love end? Would they have no option but to normalise a relationship that society was in fact incapable of accepting as something normal? Would they not turn into the mirror image of those grotesque homosexual couples where one does all the cooking and the other always goes to the market to do the shopping? Where the two lovers resemble each other in their attitudes, in their way of doing things, even in their facial expressions, to the point where they become two pathetic replicas of one and the same unbearable imaginary male, emasculated and effeminate? In the course of time would they not become two hysterical androids, forever on the point of butting in every time the other spoke, with that facial skin that is a bit too smooth and taut and tanned, and that hair that is a bit too perfect the way it hides thinning spots? Would they ever manage to accept growing older with manly dignity, not just where their bodies were concerned, but where their very dreams, and thus their love for each other, were concerned?

Leo did not have the answers to all these questions. But he was sure of one thing. He did not want to live in the same house, in the same city as Thomas. He wanted to go on being a separate lover, he wanted to go on dreaming his love, and he did not want to get stuck in everyday life. If they lived together they would become caricatures of each other, like two obscene, face-lifted twins in a Berlin cabaret. He was quite sure that he loved Thomas, and that he wanted him to be his for the rest of his life, right to the very end. But not in his room. How could he get Thomas to understand this without hurting him, without offending him?

The break, when it came, was sudden and unexpected, even if things had been working up to it for days of indifference and listlessness, shabby togetherness and quarrels. Every day the same scene played itself out. They would quarrel and then they would make it up. Each time it happened things became just a little bit more compounded, until suddenly there was an inevitable overflowing of hatred and violence. Thomas left Milan.

This time Leo did not go with him to the train. He got to his feet just to shut the door of the apartment with a double turn of the key. Thomas, waiting outside on the landing for the elevator, must have heard the clatter of the lock and Leo imagined how mortally offended he would be. He felt mean and ridiculous. But deep down he was glad to be on his own. He turned on the stereo, took the phone off the hook and lay back on the sofa with a bottle of Calvados. He took a long swig. He could smell the autumnal scent of apples. It made him think of France and the trips he had made with Thomas – trips they would perhaps never make again.

For several weeks there was no news of Thomas. Leo, for his part, did not try to call him or write to him. Every now and then, in the dead of night, the telephone rang. Leo answered, but there was no voice at the other end. But he could sense that there was somebody there, hunched over the mouthpiece, refusing to say anything. So sometimes he would whisper a 'good night' to that silent caller before he hung up.

In the end he felt lucid enough to write Thomas a long letter. In it he said he missed him, that he still loved him, and that Thomas must be strong enough to accept the way their relationship was developing. Because he found himself slipping into the realm of pathos, a condition that Leo considered in order between distant lovers, but certainly not appropriate for this moment of clarification and adjustment, he decided instead to send Thomas Joe Jackson's 'We Can't Live Together', with the words: 'Why can't you be just more like me or me like you, and why can't one and one just add up to two. But we can't live together, and we can't stay apart.'

Thomas wrote back by return post: 'Sometimes I feel terribly ill at ease and I wander round the apartment feeling incredibly frustrated. You know, I've always been terrified of not keeping it together and I thought with you close by everything would be easier. Other days it's quite different: I feel that everything becomes amazingly natural, I feel that feelings, pleasures and everything in the world that's indescribable and wonderful manages to find form, while I'm playing the piano or composing. At other times, like now, for example, after a kind of emotional breakdown caused by your letter and listening to the tape, I tell myself: keep cool . . . just accept what's happened to you for what it is. Dear one, other times you come into my thoughts, and it seems as if someone is stopping me from thinking about you, from seeing you, you for example, you who always give me the go-ahead about how to think about you, so many times a day, not too intensely, adagio, lento, piano, and then stop, really stop. I feel like I'm a toy train forever being shunted from one track to another, in bursts, with a rhythm that's always uneven and full of disorder. Like I'm choking on impatience and restlessness.'

Another page, written with a different pen, read: 'To get back to us, every so often we find ourselves not having any trust in anything. People change in your mind into puppets and you can make them move the way you want. Or rather, it's your fear that moves these puppets, this little theatre inside you, in a scenario that's already been worked out, that culminates in your favourite ending: disappearance from the face of the earth. So by being aware of all this, I find myself turning you into a sadistic puppet master and I hate you. But then you come back and console me. You understand me and love me; and then I look at your eyes, in a photo, and they are as comforting as they were the last time. I make a pact with the devil. I want your eyes, all over again and at any price. I smoke a cigarette to seal the pact, but then, my darling, I discover to my horror that the devil is none other than you.'

Leo answered this and other letters very thoroughly and thoughtfully. He spent every morning writing. In those letters, for him as well as for Thomas, there was a sense of continually going back over their relationship, with references to and memories of their journeys together, their mutual friends, and various other details described in their private jargon. But what he felt to be even more important was that, as letter followed letter, he and Thomas were gradually working out a new code of words appropriate for their love. During the months of this first major separation when both were somehow 'present', what required the greatest effort was keeping the possibility of words open, the possibility of contact and discussion, by avoiding the pitfall of being dragged down by boredom and indolence and indifference. In a certain sense, with their letters they were changing the course of their desire to be lovers. They were diverting it from the realm of sexuality to the realm of language. As yet they did not realise it, but in sending their letters to each other they were still making love, every day. They were still creating a tangible fruit of their union, albeit one made of paper and words. But perhaps for this very reason their love was more durable and more stable. Their letters expressed not just what was in their heart, in their imagination, and in their intellect and mind. Above all their letters became a record of their life together, like two scribes passionately committing it to paper, for the sake of History. So their letters progressed from being love letters to being records of a kind of evolution. From this, they then grew as if calcified, like white blocks of granite, turning into things found in an archaeological excavation of their impossible, but real, attempt at love. Their togetherness began to put behind it the emptiness of some desperate, nameless brand of love. It also started to write its own autobiography. As a result, it was being born and starting to exist no longer just for them, but for others, even more so. For they were two small, finite entities, Leo and Thomas, who would soon vanish from the world along with all their friends and all the people they had ever known, and then they would turn back into nothing more than a handful of dry, crumbling bones. They were searching for the right words to talk of all this, and this force and stress of writing, which had something to do with music and lamentation and devoutness, was the only moment when they could see themselves attached to other people, when their circumscribed life could attain the boundaries of the epic.

Day in day out, and regardless of the inconvenience of the distance between them, their relationship was working itself out and, paradoxically enough, heading towards a new balance. The two words, but with a significance that seemed to Leo to be as full and adequate as a well worked out concept – the tiny phrase that he found himself writing in one of his letters was 'separate rooms'. And he explained to Thomas that, with him, what he wanted was a relationship based on proximity, a relationship that involved belonging to each other, but not possessing each other. He explained he was happier to be on his own, but at the same time he thought of Thomas as his preferred lover, the favourite partner in a perennial engagement. He explained that they should not be afraid of their solitude, that, rather, they should experience it as the most complete fruit of their love, because, essentially, even being apart, they belonged to one another and still loved each other. He explained that they would spend the spring and summer of every year travelling together, and that in the winter they would each work on their own projects. He explained that it was a difficult choice, above all a different choice, but that in his heart he, Leo, knew he could not handle it any other way. Last of all he explained that he would be faithful to 'separate rooms' until his death.

At this point Leo felt so strong and reassured about his love for Thomas – he was suddenly seeing himself in perspective and no longer in the flatness of the present – that decided to spend a few days with him in Berlin. He took presents for Thomas: pipe tobacco, a pale grey sweater, and two copies of the same novel so that they could both read it together.

When he walked through customs into the international arrivals hall he felt slightly nervous, and impatient to take Thomas in his arms again. At passport control he had thought of that sweetest of sensations – the one he was currently living – of landing in a different, distant city with the certainty that someone had come to meet him, that there was a car in the parking lot ready to whisk him away, and that before very long he would be able to sink into a sofa in the peace and quiet of an apartment that was scented with fir or beechwood. And happiness seemed to him to have to do with being able to take a silent look around at the place where the person you love is living. But Thomas was not there to meet him. Leo waited near the arrivals board, becoming more and more worried, then he started to pace about, just a few yards up and down to begin with, as if he were afraid of getting lost, then further and further, going as far as the bar and the shops and the check-in counters. Thomas was nowhere to be found. He tried telephoning him, but there was no answer. He finally found somewhere to sit down, put his presents on the adjacent seat, and stared at his hands, waiting.

As he had done so many times before, he had imagined in his mind's eye seeing Thomas roaming around the wide corridors of the airport, wearing a shabby pullover, pipe in hand, with that shy look on his face, always a bit on edge in the thick of a crowd. He had imagined himself emerging through the automatic doors and their eyes meeting straightaway. He would have smiled and winked, blushing with emotion, and Thomas would have come towards him, cleaving a way through the crowd, to hug him and take his luggage. But it was all part of some dream. Leo doggedly imagined those moments of his life as if in a song: distance, an embrace, contact between faces and a light kiss to say hello. He kept on thinking that love was the wonderful holiday of his life. A weekend to be spent together with the loved one, by candlelight, with a landscape to gaze at and some good rum to drink. Perhaps 'separate rooms' was the illusion, perhaps it was just a bit too tourist-like, that his idea of love was only in songs and books. But what other kind of love could there be?

Thomas arrived at the run, dashing across the now deserted concourse, half an hour late. Leo spotted him some way off and got to his feet, breaking into a smile. Walking at a brisk pace, Thomas shook his head by way of apology, and Leo, with all his packages, felt like a Christmas tree after the festivities were over: pathetic and out of it.

'I had a hell of a job parking,' Thomas said, hugging him.

Leo sensed that he was embarrassed as he stiffened at their touch. 'Don't worry. Let's get out of here.'

As they drove away from the airport Leo started to feel uneasy. He pulled his coat tightly around him as if he wanted to hide. So as not to give the impression that he was suffering, he asked Thomas for news of this and that every so often, and which way they were going. They both uttered sentences that could only be answered with a yes or a no. They were not questions: they were state-ments of a shared feeling of malaise.

Unlike Leo, Thomas seemed calm and composed, or at least he gave the impression of managing to handle his awkwardness. When they stopped at traffic-lights he turned his head and stroked Leo's hand. Leo felt more and more ill at ease. He could grasp who he was sitting next to. It was Thomas, of course, his friend Thomas. But he still could not be sure. He sensed that he was aloof, apart, a person whom months of separation had completely changed. He recognised the smell of him, his voice, the affectionate gestures of his hands, that particu-lar way he had of looking at him and smiling at him, but there was too much Thomas in what he was seeing. He was no longer seeing the Thomas of 'Thomas-and-Leo', as he had once. This impossibility of recognising him made him afraid. His first instinct would have been to get out of the car, hail a cab and go right back to where he had come from. Be on his own and think about what was happening. Regain his balance. Maybe they had stayed apart too long. In those other years they had seen each other every month. Even if it meant tiring journeys, they never let more than three weeks between meetings. And they rarely met for less than four or five days. But now, after all the months that had elapsed, and all those letters, they really were two different people. They had not changed, they had simply been replaced. The picture that Leo had in his mind's eye was one of two travellers who, at a certain point, had got off the same train. And by some accident or coincidence they had boarded two parallel trains both heading in the same direction, very, very slowly. And then, just like that, the tracks had started to diverge, one heading left and the other right. In a way they were still travelling together, but they were picking up speed and all of a sudden a huge space opened up between the two trains, a space that could not be bridged, and each one of them found himself alone, travelling along his own itinerary with the image of that detour still in their mind, and the last carriages disappearing from view behind a hill. And the speed increasing. Nobody can get off, and nobody can turn back.

Leo suddenly thinks: 'It's over.'

That evening, in Thomas's apartment, it took every ounce of determination he had, and even his childish stupidity that refused to comprehend the change that had taken place – perhaps precisely because he happened to get wind of the new situation before anybody else – to say to himself: 'He's still mine. And everything's going to turn out for the best.' It took all his courage to stretch out a hand and caress him, lying on the bed beside him, as if not there, perhaps sad, and closed off. Then Leo avoided

191

asking him what was happening, pretending, as he had on so many other occasions in the months before they parted, that the absence of harmony between them must be due to tiredness, to the distance between them, and to the fact that they had got out of the habit of being affectionate with each other, and thus not to any real disaster. So Leo drank a little to pluck up courage, and then he kissed Thomas. And he buried his face in Thomas's chest and felt awkward and ashamed, because Thomas was just lying there motionless. Then at last he felt the pressure of Thomas's hand resting on his head and stroking his hair. At that moment he lost his self-control and started sobbing. He moved away from Thomas, hid his face in his hands, curled up and wept.

Thomas let him give vent to his tears. He pressed his hand hard against Leo's face and Leo seized it and kissed it and used it to dry his eyes. It was the only physical contact between them and, for Leo, it was too much.

'I don't know what's happening to me,' he sobbed.

Thomas tried not to catch his eye and said, as if he were thinking of something quite different: 'Sometimes a certain type of caress cuts deeper than a razor. I love you Leo. But you're the one who's come here, and it was up to you to make the first move. Sometimes there are terrible moments when you push me away. And others when, just as unexpectedly, you want my company.

'You're unpredictable and I can't follow your moods. One minute you're here, then you're gone. And when you want me, because you've put the absurd idea into your own head that I should be on call, you arrive as if nothing at all happened during all those months. And I have to get used to the idea of you all over again. I have to love you, and then I have to stop loving you when you can't stand it any more. I have to be here for you, and then I have to vanish. If I need you just once, and come looking for you, and if my needing you doesn't coincide with the moment when you cry out for me, then I'm trespassing. And I can't do anything about it. I have either to go away or put up with being mistreated. I have to put up with your scorn and your irony. Your insults. Leo, why don't you come to terms with your heart and accept the fact that you love me?'

He spoke slowly, trying hard to find the right words. Leo sensed that Thomas's outburst was not something frivolous or haphazard. It was a part he had learnt after months and months of rehearsals. It was sincere and genuine, and at the same time it was too precise, too worked out to be mere response. Every word that Thomas uttered had a sense of tangible pain that had given birth to that word – an effort of concentration and reflection. And Leo felt even worse. Why was he humiliating this young man? How could he allow himself to ruin his life like this? He was removing the joy from a love story, from living together with the person he loved. He was tearing him apart by involving him in the twisted mess of his own character. He looked at Thomas with no enthusiasm, and it struck him that he was entirely to blame.

Leo's sobbing gave way to a state of feeling absent, a dazed state of bewilderment. His face felt drenched and red-hot, his eyes swollen and his arms lifeless. His legs felt cold. He was shivering. Thomas took the duvet and covered him with it. He rolled a cigarette, lit it and took a few puffs. He put the cigarette between Leo's lips. Then he sat down at the foot of the bed with his head leaning against the edge. He waited until Leo had stopped smoking, stubbed out the butt in the ashtray and lay close to him in the bed, kissing him. 'I needed to see you so badly,' Leo murmured, pressing himself so hard against Thomas that it almost hurt.

At around four in the morning, after searching for hours, they finally found one another in that perfect point of pleasure and affection that they had both already known before. They thought they might have lost it forever. Having found it again, they decided to go out. Thomas was famished and there was nothing to eat in the apartment. Leo said he felt like having a walk, and being among people for a bit. 'There's a Turkish place that stays open all night,' Thomas said. 'It's not far. Brioches and coffee. Okay?'

Leo nodded his approval. He hugged him again, for a long time. They chatted away for a while, as happens between even the most quarrelsome and melancholy of lovers. They were tired of being aloof with each other, so they held hands or linked arms round their waists. There was a slight problem, even if an amusing one, when it came to slipping their hands inside each other's clothes. They were like two drunks in the latter stages of getting sozzled: lurching about, unsteady on their legs, full of mirth and all over the place. They laughed for no reason. They pinched and nipped each other or slapped each other on the back, pretended to put on a trial of strength, tumbled to the ground with their legs in the same pair of jeans. Leo said he felt like a happy fool; he said it was like

194

a moment of enlightenment, and he was approaching the state of consciousness of an eastern sage. Thomas agreed that at that hour, after everything that had happened, they were both truly weird.

They went on joking in the car and the situation between them was quite the opposite to what it had been a few hours earlier. If no words happened to pass between them, their silence was full of tenderness. It was a gentle, affectionate silence – the silence of a nestful of sleeping cubs. They reached the café and Thomas started voraciously eating the toy-like Turkish sweets, apple fritters and brioches. Leo drank very strong tea and ate out of Thomas's plate. They were bent over their table in a corner, not bothering to look around them, quite indifferent to their surroundings. More than once a friend of Thomas's came over to them, and slapped Thomas's shoulder to distract him from his plateful of food and say hello: Thomas giggled, introduced Leo as 'an Italian friend', but with such tenderness and confidence in his voice that the others understood the situation and Leo returned their hellos and felt proud at this acknowledgement.

They left shortly before six, when the metro starts to run again and young people take over the stations in a rush to get home. But they did not go to sleep right away. Thomas took Leo on a long drive towards Kreuzberg, and then in the direction of the Wilmersdorf lakes. Leo asked if he could drive. Thomas let him.

'Where d'you want to go?' he asked.

'Don't know,' Leo said.

'Okay. But watch out for the cops.'

They drove around for more than an hour. To start with Thomas laid his head across Leo's lap and dropped off to sleep. Leo could feel his regular breathing and started to rock him to sleep. Looking down he could see Thomas's face, concentrating on the act of sleeping, his nostrils widening, his hair tousled and hanging long over his neck. He needed to think and move as if, by driving through the deserted city, it was easier to access his thoughts, and make them clearer.

During the night, in fact just a few hours earlier, Thomas had said to him: 'You want to keep me at a safe distance so you can write to me. If I lived with you, you wouldn't write those letters of yours. And you wouldn't be able to think of me like a character in your stage production. There must be something not quite right, in me too, if I accept to love you on these terms … Sometimes I think of you as a vulture. And you scare me. It's as if you needed fresh flesh every day to feed on. To get it you shred and tear and rip. You don't wonder who your victim is, or if your victim is a friend, or loves you or is indifferent to you. There's greed in the way you are with the people who live around you, and it scares me. And it scares me all the more because I know that deep down in you there is only genuine goodness.'

He had to think about all this. He felt strange, vulnerable, a bit jet-lagged like after a long intercontinental flight. But he was happy to have found Thomas again. More and more they both shared one common destiny. Leo was quite sure of this. He woke Thomas up with a gentle nudge to tell him he was lost. Thomas took the wheel again and they went home.

During the days that followed they planned a trip to Dresden. Thomas saw to getting the visas they needed while Leo got in touch with one or two magazines to see about placing an article with them. They left by train and when they got back to Berlin, three days later, they were even more tightly and solidly together.

When the time came for Leo to leave, for the umpteenth time, neither of them had grown accustomed to this brutal curtailment of their times together. Thomas secretly slipped a note into Leo's pocket. Leo did not discover it until the following day, back in Milan. It read: 'I'm listening to our song, while you're getting dressed, in the other room and every so often you come in and look at me and ask me what I can possibly be listening to that's so moving. I don't hear what you're saying, but I understand. Everything is so strong that it's tiring to organise words in the right order. Last night, when I went home, I wasn't afraid, either of leaving or of moving on, or of stopping myself from thinking about you. All I felt was a strength which was pushing me on, forward, like surf on an ocean wave. I wanted to explore, and show you the way and then change directions, because even you were feeling dizzy from my eternal seasickness. I hope I managed it. Now you must leave. It all seems shrouded by a cloak of indifference. My senses are concentrated on preserving my memories of you and the sound of your voice. I'm withdrawing into myself. It's a process that will take a few hours and I'll come out of it again when you're just a tiny indecipherable speck inside another tiny speck, far away from the sky over Berlin.'

The 'separate rooms' strategy seemed to develop, in the ensuing months, in a way that Leo managed to keep control of, and in a way that did not make him feel that he was squandering too much of himself and his own energy. He found time to write and work. Lodged in his mind was a person whom he loved, someone he could hear at the other end of the telephone, someone to whom he was devoting everything he did, someone whom he desired and wrote letters to. He was quite sure that his love for Thomas had reached its zenith. It could go no higher. It could merely change by adopting different embodiments and figures.

He was pleased that he had managed to put a thousand miles and more between their two respective bedrooms, a distance which, incidentally, neither of them felt was so huge that it might hamper their relationship. Thomas, on the other hand, had cleverly and stubbornly managed to introduce a third person into their 'separate rooms'. More importantly, he had also managed to persuade Leo to accept this new situation, in the name of their love.

It certainly was not easy. When Leo got to know that Thomas was living with someone else he was furious. He felt betrayed and, worse still, humiliated. But Thomas would not budge: 'You want to live on your own, Leo. But I want to live with the person I love.'

'This means it's all over between us,' Leo said.

Thomas did not answer. Then, in a mortified tone of voice, he said: 'We've got to talk about it as soon as we see each other again. I can't talk about it like this.'

Leo reacted violently. During the days that followed he wrote letters almost every day in which he railed against

198

Thomas, accusing him of wanting to destroy him for some wretched business about sex. He refused to understand that Thomas was missing him too much, and suffering as a result. The third person was not a substitute for Leo. He was just a person with whom Thomas shared the same idea of love. Or rather she . . . Thomas was living with a twenty-year-old woman. With her Thomas felt happy, and confident in the future, whereas with Leo there was non-stop arguing, which he had to put up with and, above all, put up with too much pain. And the fact that Leo did not understand that he was still the only man in his life made him feel even worse about it all. One day he wrote to him that he was not going to open any more letters that Leo sent him; he would destroy them all because he knew, now, how offensive their contents would be, and how insulting to Susann, too, even though Leo did not even know her. He also said that both Susann and Leo ought to consider themselves lucky because they knew for sure what they both wanted, whereas he, Thomas, could not make up his mind. He was still in love with Leo, but he was also in love with Susann. He would have to give up one or other of them, but he did not know how to go about it. Susann would live with him and Leo would not. That was why he had decided to do without Leo.

Leo went on telephoning Thomas and writing to him, asking if he could come and see him. They did finally meet, in the spring. And Thomas found Leo so genuinely in pain that he took pity on him. The evening before, they had met, formally, in a half-empty restaurant on the outskirts of the city. Leo had trouble talking to Thomas.

He kept his eyes lowered and muttered. Thomas told him that he could not go on with Leo: he was happy with Susann. However, he did not forget what they had meant to each other and once a bit of time had passed they would make peace again. Yet, as he spoke, he had the sensation that Leo was thinking about other things and that it was all too painful for him. They said their goodbyes, squeezing each other's hand, Leo in his car and Thomas waiting for a taxi to take him back to the hotel where Susann was waiting for him. But the next day he called on the telephone and said: 'I've got rid of Susann. I'm coming over to your place. Let's have a holiday. We both need one.'

They set off for Spain. They were in love. But there was still a shadow that fell between them. And when Thomas strayed away from Leo to buy little pieces of handcrafted jewellery, knowing full well whom they were for, Leo turned glum because Thomas had a life in which he would never play a part. With time, and by dint of the love that they still felt for each other, he started to accept this strange three-way relationship. One day, in a train, in a crowded compartment, Leo had said to him in a melancholy tone: 'I've always wanted everything, Thomas. And I've always had to make do with just anything.'

Thomas had not answered. He had looked straight into Leo's eyes and suddenly started crying quietly. His wide eyes were bright and Leo felt confused. He took his hand and realised that despite the fact that they had both strenuously done everything possible over the years to complicate each other's lives, they were madly in love with each other. And they would go on being in love all their life.

So on a magnificent February day when you can already sense the onset of spring, when Leo looks at the road map of Europe to decide which direction to head off in in the car, he thinks straightaway of Thomas and experiences an indefinable combination of satisfaction and resentment – satisfaction and pleasure, because his story is still going on, it exists and as such it soothes him; resentment, because he has to accept the fact that Thomas is living with Susann. The balance and harmony between him and Thomas now has to pass through this person whom Leo does not know and does not want to know, but whom he has to reckon with when he wants to see Thomas. A spectre, but not for Thomas of course, flitting over their separate beds. Basically all three of them are alone. No one entirely possesses anybody else, but all three belong to each other. Leo's life involves Thomas, just as Thomas's involves Leo. Each one of them is responsible for the lives of the other two, regardless of the fact that there is separateness and distance between them. Leo and Thomas are in love, at peace with each other, at the precise moment when they have sensed how impossible their love is. They love one another because they have already taken leave of each other.

So when Leo leafs through the atlases scattered around the apartment, looking for a destination for their next journey together, he thinks that he has invented a kind of love in which he believes, a kind of love which he is not demanding too much of. Just as happened with his religious sentiments, restricted to a space not of truth but of questing, so now with love. He feels conscious of the fact that he will never find peace and that, for people like him, nothing will ever be enough. Keeping these worlds close to his heart, not letting his anxiety destroy them, keeping them apart and at the same time keeping them close to his own life. Roaming from one country to the next. This is his lot.

This moment, with maps spread out on the parquet floor of the living-room, on the sofas or on his study desk, is the last recollection of peace remaining before the catastrophe. The last moment of calm before the telephone rings and it is Thomas's father telling him there is nothing more to be done, Thomas is going.

After his trip to the United States he stays in Milan for a while, on his own. He does not feel like seeing his friends, he does not talk to them on the telephone, and he does not answer letters that arrive for him. He needs to think about everything that happened to him in Washington. He needs time to digest the impact that that act is having on his solitude. He realises that he will have to accept it as part of himself, something that might also never happen again, in those times and in those conditions, but something that has brought to the surface of his consciousness the thing that he has always denied: namely, that he is riddled not just with goodness, as Thomas always maintained, but also with guilt. On the other hand, denying himself any chance of a new affair, any chance of a new love, as he has been doing for years now, is driving him crazy. He is gloomy, his thoughts dark, he is prone to nervous fits, unable to sleep properly, and he tends to be depressed every day. And towards the end of the year, when he casually tots up three years without Thomas, he realises that he has never really made love with anyone since. Sex has been just with one night stands. Then he realises that by renouncing love – and in a way this attitude has been forced upon him – he is dying, he is becoming more and more aloof from other people, confined to a rotten, barren place from which it is harder and harder to escape.

He feels an unresolved lump of bitterness and loathing. He could easily let go of himself and become violent. He sees the past as an endless series of wrongs that have been inflicted on him. He feels betrayed as if everyone had abused him, exploiting his name, his friendship, his knowledge and his generosity. He thinks that for years all he has done is grant requests made by other people, as if everybody was forever wanting something from him, whereas he has never asked or laid claim to anything whatsoever. The response to all this is a desire for revenge which focuses on every person he has known or met in the past few years. At times a sudden feeling of surprise comes over him, as he absent-mindedly looks at the television, when he discovers that for a whole couple of hours he has been thinking of nothing else bar the orchestration of a perfect crime.

The more serious fact is that his renunciation is making his body more and more unknowable and alien to him. Chastity is a mystical virtue for those who have chosen it; and perhaps the superhuman use of one's sexuality. For Leo this forced abstinence is nothing other than one more torture which is turning his natural need for physicality, touching, caresses, and the sight of another naked body into an obsession. So when he looks at himself in the bathroom mirror, as he gets out of the shower or shaves, it is with a devastating bitterness that he discovers his body, a body that was once slim and lithe and that is now more and more bloated and plump – rotund like a baby, or a china Buddha; or perhaps, if he is really cruel, flabby and soft like the body of a eunuch.

By losing the dimension of his body, by no longer being able to measure reality by a yardstick of sexual maturity – because it is only in this sense that man is exactly the measure of anything else – he finds himself suffering from dizzy spells, banging his elbows against things and knocking into things around the apartment. To take hold of an ashtray he unconsciously deploys the strength required to lift a whole piece of furniture. To take a sheet of paper he uses the energy needed to move a chair. Things drop from his hands and break. Everything he does becomes like a hostile action. Objects slip through his fingers. If things have become this rotten it is also because Leo has always found it easier, for his own character, to give up rather than plod on, to fade out rather than keep going. He has had plenty of opportunity, but after a while he has always preferred to yield to defeat, reckoning it to be much less complicated, and better for his health, to be content with a symbolic victory than to lower his guard. By refusing to play the game again with other people, by postponing any desire to do with physical bargaining, by likening the ideal of 'making love' to a furtive, hasty matter of sexual barter, the love act becomes something mythical and very remote once again, exactly like when he was a young boy. To such a point that often, when he sees two people kissing in the street, the sight of them annoys him deep down, provoking that feeling of bewilderment, jealousy, admiration and envy that a beggar from the Third World might experience when faced with a display of western opulence; or a poor handicapped wretch might feel as he watches the performance of a handsome Olympic athlete. Once more, paradise is always for the others.

At such times, as a defence, he often bursts out cursing, saying things like 'What the hell am I looking at!' and even more often, as he walks along in a crowd, he says out loud: 'I don't believe it! It can't be true!' This attitude seems all the more unacceptable to him because he has always regarded himself as tolerant, uninhibited, ready to see both sides of things, and even ready to accept other people's reasons for things. Now, this resurgence of moralism and this rigid behaviour locks him into a permanent state of muttering and mumbling, a state of suffocating grumbling aimed at everything and everyone, that seems to know no bounds. When he takes a more lucid look at himself, one morning when he has miraculously woken up in what seems to be a good mood, he sees himself as a character from a Goldoni play: an old Po Valley yokel. At such times he even manages a smile.

It is in one such moment, suspended somewhere between self-mockery and self-pity, that Leo accepts Rodolfo's invitation to stay in his house in southern Tuscany for a while. After a few days of total isolation Leo asks Rodolfo if he can come and stay with him in Florence. Rodolfo interprets this as an important step in Leo's return to normality.

'I'll throw a party for you,' he says. 'You have no idea how many people would like to see you again.'

'Are you serious?' Leo asks sardonically.

Rodolfo leaps to his feet and raises his voice: 'That's all over with, Leo. You better believe it. You've already paid enough dues, if that's what you were trying to do. There are so many beautiful men around who'd love nothing more than to shack up with someone like you. Someone who's got time for them, someone who'll travel with them and take them to the theatre and get them into any place they want—'

'Seems like I'd be a good match, eh?' Leo interrupts him.

Rodolfo does not answer right away. He knows that Leo would not expect it from him. He knows he may hurt Leo, but he is beginning to understand that this is precisely what Leo has been looking for for a while now in other people. 'Thomas wasn't a big thing, Leo,' he explains. 'An ordinary bloke. A musician heading straight for a dead-end career. He didn't know who he was, and he didn't know what he wanted either. Can't you see, you're spending more time trying to forget about him than you ever really spent with him. It could go on like this for twenty years. A whole lifetime together. For Christ's sake, Leo, all it was was a three-year flirt! No more no less. You lived together for two months, or maybe three, or five at the most. And you're wasting your life away for the sake of a few nights you spent with a stranger?'

'It wasn't just three years,' Leo answers calmly. 'I spent more than half my adult sexual life with him. So I can tell you that in this case it's not just a matter of years. Thomas was everything to me. He was ideal.'

Rodolfo looks hard at Leo, shaking his head: 'He was not the right man for you. You're not doing yourself any good making that mistake.'

Leo's voice sounds slightly cracked: 'What mistake?'

Rodolfo flops down into an armchair. He lets out a long sigh: 'The fact is, Leo, he's dead. And you're not. That's why he's not the right man for you.'

Neither of them says anything for a few minutes. They do not find it in them to raise their eyes and look at each other. Rodolfo knows he has hurt Leo and Leo is aware of the fact that his friends have been talking about him for years now, his friends have been forming their opinions about him and, most probably, thinking about how to solve the problem of a partner for him. He feels embarrassed, locked into his own silence. Rodolfo seems far away to him, unable to understand him. But on the other hand, has Leo ever really done anything to let Rodolfo – or any other friend for that matter – really understand him? If the truth be told, he has won the arduous struggle to overcome his own solitude. He has discovered that he can survive in his own company. As a guru might put it, he has turned an eye inwards to travel far in what might be called 'Leo's world'. But in so doing he has closed himself off to other people. By making himself capable of surviving alone, within his own self, he has simply exchanged death responses for life responses. No love, no passion, no friendship, no contact with the outside world, except for the little tasks of day-to-day life. This had seemed to him to be a wise solution, and it had suited him well as the years went by. His casualness with his friendships, even those which were closer to his heart than most, was dictated by the fact that he was focusing in on himself and could not be deflected for any reason whatsoever. Now he realises that while he has forgotten about other people, other people still remember him, still talk about him and wonder what he is doing with his life. And this gives him a feeling of being hemmed in. It is as if he had no code of conduct with Rodolfo now. They are offering to throw a party for him, with a few men and a little high society. Nothing out of the ordinary. Things people do for other people. He can find nothing better to do than react by taking umbrage. Because the real truth is that Rodolfo's offer has offended him. And he is treating Rodolfo with disdain.

'How could Rodolfo possibly imagine anything so frivolous, for me?' he asks himself. Then he realises that Rodolfo cannot do any different because Rodolfo does not know, because Leo has kept him at arm's length, Rodolfo and all the other people who are fond of him. Then he feels that it is probably time to get back to life, time to acknowledge the death responses for what they really are and the life responses for the good things that they might bring him.

At times, life gives rise to semantic muddles like this.

People adapt to them and go on living, forgetting the fact that the odd sign has changed: the same things, the same gestures, the same people, but everything going in the opposite direction. Data processing is the same, but the sign before, the one above or below the zero, has changed. At times, though, people manage to work out something essential, even from the darkest disaster: the idea of a new arrangement. A position, in the world, that does not tend towards the peace and quiet of the infant, but which accepts to risk itself in the unknown that is the present. At other times people proceed merely by inertia, forgetting that this just tends to dim their energy and fade out towards a dead centre. And in some ways Leo has reached this point, this dead centre. He needs a new input, a new charge, he needs to believe wholeheartedly that life is still carrying on. He must finally move on towards the separation between who is alive and who is dead. He must get rid of the vulture in him. Because if one thing is certain, it is that for all these years he has kept himself alive by eating off the mortal remains of Thomas, slaking his thirst by drinking his blood, sating his appetite on his butchered flesh like any insatiable predator before a carcass in the bush.

They are telling him that Thomas is dead. And what if Thomas were really dead? Is this what they want to get him to understand? That it is time now to leave Thomas to his own fate? But if he and Thomas had just one fate between them, how could he leave him? Have three years, or four, of this unbearable mourning served no purpose then? Have they not brought him some comfort? Why, then, has he not managed to get rid of his pain and his grief yet, why has he not managed to free himself of all that? He has managed to survive, to keep going, that's for sure, but at what price?

Then Leo wonders if by trying to contain his own grief in a personal place that is inaccessible to others, and by distilling that grief drop by drop in solitude, he has made the final distilling of his mourning something impossible to achieve. By depriving himself of social activities and by not taking part in any kind of group, he has remained in a passive anxiety zone. By refusing to socialise, he has deprived himself of that element of purification that marks any and every public expression of a feeling, even the spasmodic mourning for the loss of one's one partner. Precisely for this reason he was unable to show his grief, just as he had realised during that Good Friday procession in his home town. Because no society would acknowledge a mourning such as his as real. Nor, as a result of that, would it have the appropriate social rituals for a tragedy that has still not been officially recognised: in a word, what anthropologists call 'the mourning of the heart', as opposed to bureaucratic mourning.

So to accept discussion of it, as he is doing indirectly with Rodolfo, is a way of overcoming it. Maybe he should accept Rodolfo's invitation even if the immediate feeling of aversion he has would seem to rule out any such thing. So he plucks up courage and says: 'I'd like it better if you'd organise a dinner, something more intimate than a party.'

Rodolfo smiles. He already has his address-book in his hand. He dials a number. 'I know two Madisons you'll like. I've been keeping them on the back-burner for months.'

The restaurant Rodolfo has chosen for his production is a rather pretentious place in the middle of Florence, in the converted stables of a Renaissance mansion. He has reserved a small room with frescoes on the vaulted ceiling and a restored tiled floor that still shows the patina of time. There is barely room for the table for four and the stand for the wine bucket. First they met at Gilli's, at nine o'clock, for a glass of sparkling wine. That way no one would have to wait at the restaurant. Leo is ill at ease, but Rodolfo handles the introductions with his usual tactfulness and his over-professional expertise. Even at first glance, the two other men definitely belong to the Madison category, Florentine variety. In other words, the American college type, good family, with a tight, athletic physique and dazzling conversation. They arrive on a huge Yamaha motorcycle and park in the square opposite the bar. The driver, Ruben, is about twenty, with long fair hair, a full mouth, light-coloured eyes, not very tall, but solidly built. He is wearing a black leather jacket, jeans and black English shoes. Round his neck he has a scarf with tiny white dots. The other guy, Eugenio, is a tall, lean young man, with brown wavy hair and an ancient, delicate look about him. His eyes are greyish. He is wearing a blue blazer, a red-and-blue small-check shirt, a pair of jeans and suede boots. They walk towards the bar taking off their helmets. Rodolfo leaves Leo and goes to meet them. The conversation in the restaurant is none too thrilling.

Rodolfo orchestrates the topics skilfully, with a keen eye for anything that will involve all four of them, but it is not that easy. The best thing would be to talk about a movie or a show, but he is worried that the Madisons might say the wrong thing and annoy Leo. What is more, they have already talked about the friends they have in common, and here, too, things never really warmed up. When there is a lull in the conversation, someone quickly says something and addresses Leo. At the beginning of the meal Leo interpreted this as pleasant, but now he feels it is hypocritical. He imagines that Rodolfo rehearsed the two Madisons in advance, and asked them to be attentive to Leo. Leo feels that he is being looked at with pity and perhaps even with compassion. The efforts the others make seem clumsy, because all they do is remind him of how alone he is. Even when they talk of beaches in Greece, or ski resorts, or nights in Rome or Milan, or trips to New York and the Caribbean, he feels a look of condescension coming over his face. As if he knew all about those landscapes and places already, and what he really wanted was to sit there without saying a word, just adding the odd comment out of politeness. Eugenio, in particular, the tall, lanky one, and the one he prefers, looks at him with inquisitive kindness, as if he were waiting for Leo to make some kind of move. But Leo does nothing and at the end of the meal – a meal that will stay lodged in his memory for ever somewhere between pathos and irony, as the 'widow's supper' – when he walks with the two of them back to their motorcycle to say goodbye, he feels that he has shed a great weight.

Alone with Rodolfo, and feeling guilty because of Rodolfo's offended silence, he says to him in a gentle, friendly way: 'You see, I feel like someone who has nothing to show to anyone else. A person who has no strategies or tactics or plans of action, because, in all honesty, I'm not interested in showing myself as something I'm not any more. I know I'm someone who can also be fun, someone who can be good company. But now I'd rather other people discovered it. And anyway, from now on, I can only get involved with someone who – without me lifting a finger – understands who I am behind this sad and off-putting façade. Right now I don't want to be amusing, for the simple fact that that's not the way I'm feeling. I don't want to seduce anybody. If you'll allow me, I'll wait for other people to seduce me.'

'I thought I could help you, but you don't even want to be helped. Ruben and Eugenio are two great guys. But seeing how the evening went, I don't think I'll be able to ask them again.'

Leo looks at him for a moment, shifting the bunch of keys nervously from one hand to the other: 'Yes,' he says fleetingly before he goes up to his room, 'you're right. Eugenio's a really nice guy.'

Next day, as he is flicking through the newspapers, he hears a knock at the door. The doorman hands him a package. Leo puts it on the table, thinking it is a present for Rodolfo. But the label has his name on it. He undoes the white tissue paper and discovers, in a straw basket, an array of strawberries, cherries, radishes and chilli peppers, laid out on a bed of pink rose petals. He opens the note. It is from Eugenio.

Now the smile leaves his face. He is not amused by the oddness of the bouquet of ruby-red fruit and vegetables. He wonders what it all might mean. He is unable to accept such a homage for what it is. He starts to imagine the significance of the strawberries, or the little chilli peppers from the South. All he sees is a threat. For years he has put up such defences against the catastrophe of love that when the time is ripe to start all over again, as it may be right now, he no longer knows where or how. But the problem is precisely this: why is he already putting himself in a context of love, when maybe all it is is a statement of friendship? Why does he already imagine a demand for an emotional relationship, and why does he not interpret that little basket of fruit as the ironical and amusing comment of an intelligent, sensitive young man, with exquisite taste, on the apathy that Leo displayed the evening before? His voice unsure and awkward, Leo phones to thank him.

Eugenio seems amused, confident in the way he speaks, and above all interested in Leo. The result of the 'widow's supper', was the beginning of an affectionate friendship between Leo and that young man. Some nights, after a film or an evening spent with friends, they end up in a restaurant or a bar, talking until daybreak. On other occasions they spend whole afternoons on a sofa watching video-clips and talking about music and images and cities. And when night falls they sit down by candlelight in Rodolfo's little kitchen, pulling their chairs over to the refrigerator and carry on talking, with plates on their knees and bottles of beer on the floor. When they part, they say goodbye like old pals and on the return journey by train Leo feels again the distress of leave-taking – for the first time since his affair with Thomas ended.

But Leo knows he is not in love with Eugenio. He enjoys his company, and his conversation, and his way of looking closely at him with his wonderfully wide eyes, but he desires neither Eugenio's body nor the act of love. He admires Eugenio's quick mind, and his sensitivity, as well as that sort of devotion which he has been turning his back on for months now. But he knows that he will never be in love with Eugenio. He has reached an age when it seems right and proper to balance the books. He has given love a chance and lost. Now he knows that he is not made to love one person, he is not made for sex, or for living together with another man. He only feels at peace when he is on his own, with a few close friends to look after him. What he is doing is attempting to make a family for himself, a strange family with no women or children, but a family where the bonds between members are just as strong and conscious: Rodolfo, Eugenio, Michael, are his family now.

In any event, what bestial impulse makes men seek each other out so feverishly, so brutally, to plunder each other and hurt each other by turns? What initial disaster was it that let Eros become identifiable only in the form of genital obsession and not in terms of the mutual positions of love? How many friendships has Leo seen end, brutally and painfully, because one of the two people would not give his own body to the other? Is restricting sexuality to its proper confines, and circumscribing it, perhaps not the same as giving it its natural contour?

Everyone is accusing Leo of not making love. And the first to level such an accusation, some time ago, was Leo himself. Ever since he stopped making love, his sense of social responsibility has grown weaker and virtually disappeared. As long as he turned up at discos or parties in the company of beautiful boys, surrounded by his court, he was regarded as a man riding the wave of success, and he was respected and appreciated. Now that he is on his own, now that he still goes to clubs but only to hang out in a corner sipping beer and listening in the darkness to the music going in one ear and out the other, he is no more than a worn-out castaway. But Leo is thinking that it is time to be done with the obsession of being like other people, time to stop believing that normality means not missing a single opportunity of jumping into bed with anyone who beckons. Everyone says they know what love is, but Leo thinks that the person who truly loves other people and the whole world, trees, rivers and animals, that exceptional person is the hermit. In his own way he is a monk. This is where he differs from others.

With Thomas Leo was in love with somebody like himself. He managed to love Thomas because he learnt how to suffer and how to give. But there is nothing to say that miracles recur. When he talks with Eugenio he becomes more and more aware that there will not be another time, precisely because what he is looking for now is not a companion, but his own new place in the world. He retains his capacity for love, but he no longer invests it in another person. Rather, he invests it in what characterises the species to which he belongs. Now he is in a position to do this without committing the sin of idealism or fanaticism, because he now bears the indelible mark of the love of two people, Thomas and Leo, who have existed and whose presence he cradles tenderly in the depths of his heart. There was a time when he was wrong, a time when he found his love relationship barren and fruitless. Leo and Thomas have given birth to at least one son, even if it was painful. And this son suddenly thrust on to the world, who thinks and acts, is Leo now, aged thirty-three.

*

Eugenio follows him with the devotion of the favourite pupil who asks for nothing, demands nothing and wants nothing other than the company of his older friend. A pupil by whom Leo feels understood almost too well, like on a Sunday afternoon in November, for example, when Eugenio goes with Leo on the Rilke Walk, the trail which runs high along a clifftop ridge and links Duino castle with Sistiana. It is cold, and drizzle shrouds the outline of the crag. The sky is low and the sea below is like a motionless sheet of steel. The path zigzags along the edge of the cliff between weathered white rocks, pierced with holes by the wind as if by thousands of limestone caterpillars. The sandy ground on which they are walking is purple. The spindly branches hide bunches of bright yellow berries. Leo climbs on top of a boulder, looking sheer down to the sea. He feels the wind beneath his skin, squints away towards the horizon, but he can make out nothing except a grey backdrop streaked by air and wind and rain-charged clouds. There is no actual horizon. He cannot make out where the sea meets the sky: it is all one. Silvery shadows are reflected in the moist, salty air. On that rock, he is nothing other than an unknowable reflection being watched by the clouds and the sea. The massive castle looks like a stronghold. It soars upwards powerful and fearsome: the outpost of obscurity from which to pose answerless questions. Below, on the other side, half hidden among the limestone rocks, Eugenio is watching him, unsmiling, and without complicity. He watches him and pulls a blade of grass between his teeth. Leo realises in this very moment that Eugenio knows. He feels a strong desire, if such a thing were ever in his power to do, to bless him.

At other times Leo jokes lightheartedly about Eugenio's attitude, and hums 'Suedehead': 'Why, why do you hang around?' then he realises that behind his smiling face Eugenio is hurt. And Leo feels helpless because he does not know how to get rid of his young friend's consternation. He knows that he must keep himself at a slight remove, a slight distance from him, because he is running the risk of breaking him into small pieces. No one can be so strong that they can stand up against the shock wave of a person like Leo, or, at least, nobody who is fond of him can. He knows he must carry on behaving like those insects who drive a sting into larvae and suck on them for days and days, digest them, and feed permanently until there is nothing left except a curled up case, completely empty, a sarcophagus without a mummy inside. Then they fly around in search of other young sources of food. No, he does not want to behave with Eugenio to the point where he makes him disappear altogether, to the point where he absorbs him so completely in himself that his whole life becomes unbearable. This is why he urges him to study, to attend university lectures and courses, to take exams, to keep up his friendships with his contemporaries, and to fall in love. Leo charts Eugenio's flirtatious affairs rather as a father confessor would: he does not offer any counsel but he listens closely to whatever Eugenio has to say. Every so often he avoids Eugenio's telephone calls and visits. He disappears. Then he crops up again. Eugenio invites him to the country. Leo arrives. They hug, and listen to new records. They discuss novels that have just been published, and have discussions long into the night. Then Leo crawls into his separate bed and falls asleep, with one eye on the light filtering from Eugenio's bedroom, through the crack in the old wooden door.

Then one day in late September, he finds himself on a bus, smaller and more luxurious than a Greyhound, with reserved seats and large panoramic windows that give a wide angle view of the outskirts of Montreal, the buildings in the Olympic village, the wide trunk-roads filled with traffic that seems slow and silent, the huge bridges over the St Lawrence seaway and, above all, the vast North American sky. He watches an orange-coloured seaplane taxi across the water and take slowly to the air, like a toy or a small clockwork bird. It is four in the afternoon. He is tired from an eight-hour flight and he still has two hundred miles to travel to reach Quebec. He picks up a book but is unable to read, and when evening dims the sky and his eyes are heavy with sleep, he puts on his headphones and listens to the tapes that Eugenio has recorded for him: Morrissey, of course, and The Smiths, then Deacon Blue, Swing Out Sister, Billy Bragg, Wim Mertens . . . The bus is quiet, the violet service lights are on. He slips off his shoes, puts them to one side on the grey floor-carpet and tries to lower the back of his seat. Outside the lights of the city seem far away. Every so often a whole valley is suddenly lit up, like at the exit of a tunnel . . . There are not many passengers, and those there are he cannot see. The seats have tall backs. The rows of seats are like couchettes on a train. Then someone knocks against his legs, which he has stretched out in the central aisle. He looks up, interrupting his concentration, and sees a young man heading for the back of the bus. Then he feels his heart beat faster and he feels a very keen emotion within him, almost like a sense of gratitude. The young man, who cannot be twenty yet, has curly hair. He is wearing denim overalls and, beneath them, an ivory-coloured coarse sweater. He has joined a girl with long, sleek hair who is making a ham sandwich and opening a bottle of apple juice. They joke with each other and balance paper plates on their knees. On the ground they have several dog-eared paperbacks, their pages well thumbed and curled at the edges. Leo stares at them. The boy takes a map from a small rucksack. He opens it and props it against the back of the seat in front of him. He moves his finger over the map, tracing a route. The girl watches closely, biting into her sandwich.

They murmur things to each other in low voices. Leo remembers.

He is on a ferry boat that is slowly chugging back to Italy from Patras. It is night-time, a cold night at the end of August at sea. He is on his own, he has nothing with him to deal with a two-day journey on deck. He missed his flight in Athens and could not find a seat on any other flight to Italy. For a couple of nights he stayed in a hotel close to the airport, and went to the stand-by desk every three hours. Night and day. With his last few drachmas, he went to the bus station and boarded a coach to Patras. Here, without food or drink, he waited until nightfall for the ferry. He bought a deck ticket, the only one he could afford. When the ship weighed anchor he found himself surrounded by hundreds of young people with sleeping-bags. They all propped their rucksacks against the railings to make a bivouac for the night. He was the only person left sitting on the iron bench, solitary and far away, like a passenger from another era. He had no blankets, no rucksack, and nothing to eat. He had left Chios quite sure that he would be in Rome three hours later, but as it turned out he had been travelling now for three days, and would not be home for another three.

Near his feet some Scandinavian girls had stretched out, and beyond them a group of French boys, then German and Spanish boys, a lot of young Americans, Swiss, Brazilians, and kids from Holland and Canada. Leo could tell their nationalities not only by their bodies and their physical features, by the colour of their hair and the language they spoke – even if he could not quite tell for sure the difference between Flemish and Swedish, or Catalan and Spanish – but mainly by the flags sewn onto their rucksacks. They were like the different reverberations of the same notion of youth. Then all of a sudden, as if someone had issued a precise and incontradictable order through the loudspeaker system, they all started to rummage in their backpacks and produce paper bags and packets and wrappers, and they started to open these bundles and spread them out on their sleeping-bags. The things Leo saw emerging from those packages! Eggs, cheese, roast chicken, fruit, grapes, plums, little jars of goat yoghurt, cow yoghurt and sheep yoghurt, cherries, jars of malt, oat bran, pineapples, cartons of milk, fruit juice, orangeade, Coca-Cola, Pepsi, bottles of tonic, litres of mineral water, slices of salami, cooked

221

ham, roast beef, bacon, frankfurters, sausages, tomatoes, beetroot, sticks of celery, bunches of parsley, carrots, bell peppers, pickled onions, cottage cheese, sardines, cans of tuna fish, herring, fillets of mackerel, bream, spicy beans, creamed greens, vacuum-packed soups, consommé, and then a whole incredible array of desserts – from caramels to nougat, to brioches, to bars of chocolate, to bon-bons, to liqueur chocolates, to chocolates from Piedmont, to marzipan, to little tarts and pies, to cream puffs, to profiteroles, to apple tart, bananas, coconuts and kiwis. Thermoses and flasks full of coffee, tea, hot chocolate, camomile and mint. Leo looked on wide-eyed with amazement and incredulous at this display of abundance. Everybody ate ravenously, devouring chicken-legs and chunks of cheese that vanished into their mouths like in a cartoon. Leo remained on his bench, head and shoulders above that huge, sated crowd, pathetically small in his blue blazer, his white jeans unable to keep out the cold, and his sneakers without socks to keep his feet warm.

People rushed to and fro to the rubbish bins, with a noise like the dizzy-making flap-flapping of a flock of pigeons, yes, just as if someone had tossed a stone into the middle of that expanse of sleeping-bags and everybody had darted away. Then an orderly queue formed by the washrooms, everybody clutching toothbrushes, with towels over their shoulders. Suddenly, once again, everything stopped still and he realised that most of the young travellers were fast asleep. He saw the odd face sticking out of the covers with Walkman headphones, a few people chatting, a couple having a tender kiss, but there was a huge hush and the rolling of the ferry-boat could also seem like an old-fashioned way – precisely because it was technological – of rocking these kids to sleep. Then, for a split second, Leo experienced the intimate and moving pleasure of watching over hundreds of young slumbering charges. And it seemed possible that, by missing his connection in Athens, if he had to travel for so many days, if he had boarded this vessel and not another one, it was because he was destined to find his way to that white-painted iron bench and observe the spectacle of that youth, all contented and serene, in a way that his own youth had never been. He knew those young folk well, even if he had never met them before, even if he would probably never see any of them again, were he to live for another thousand years. Nor would they ever remember that young man sitting there as if in a theatre, with his tortoiseshell glasses, a hand-rolled cigarette endlessly smoking as it hung from his lips, protected against the cold by no more than a blue bath towel which he was endlessly pulling about his shoulders in frustration. Yet, for this reason if no other, by the light of those stars and that chill Mediterranean moon he was filled with an awareness that this was really his fate, to watch over and record. Looking at the wake of bright white foam that the ship left at its stern, spreading out like a glistening fan, frothing against the pitch black of the night, he felt somehow comforted and saw something akin to a single image of the ship and its wake and the fate of all those young and beautiful people. He could also see his own life, no longer set apart, but well positioned on the deck of something in motion – a vessel full of smiling, if spectral destinies.

*

Now, on the coach sailing silently through Quebec, he sees those two young people like contaminated presences from the thick of the bygone years of his youth. They represent the physical persistence of types and characters around whom his writing has evolved and in whom his desire is embodied. He feels protected. Or rather, he feels that his journey will have a destination. When he reaches the city and leaves the coach and turns to register their presence in his eyes one last time and thank them silently for giving him their message, he can no longer find them. Then, with a smile, he thinks that on the deck of that ship he was also perhaps in the company of angels, hungry, chattering angels to be sure, a posse of angels on a tourist trip. But at a certain moment has he not quite clearly heard the rustling of their wings?

Then one evening, he is in the long bar at the Grand Dérangement, a smart and smoky jazz club not unlike a sixties dancehall in northern Italy, the bar all shiny against a wall, almost wedged into a corner, the expanse of small tables littered with bottles of beer, the small stage, the main spotlight set in the middle of the room, a few other spots covered with coloured filters, the upright piano and the amplifiers and, on the ceiling, strings of lights. He is there along with hundreds of other people, young and old alike, the great survivors of the Beat Generation still spritely and in fighting mood, poets, writers, artists, students from the United States, England, Germany, Canada and Quebec, journalists and musicians, all gathered to celebrate the opening of the international congress on Jack Kerouac. That evening, when a blues player from California started to read from the last page of *On the Road*: 'So in America when the sun goes down and I sit on the old broken-down river pier watching the long, long skies over New Jersey and sense all that raw land that rolls in one unbelievable huge bulge over to the West Coast, and all that road going . . .', modulating his voice, pacing it, first only slightly, then with more and more cadence to let the bass come in, then the percussion, in the background, it finally became a song accompanied by the guitar. It seemed to Leo that what Kerouac had written was really the lyrics for a beautiful and tormenting jazz piece. And when the sax came in – the words were now over and the music played on, developing the imagery – he felt that all those people were, all together, celebrating a ritual which had no pomp and circumstance about it, a very simple ritual and one that was for this very reason basic: the survival of literature. The human being whom they were celebrating was not an academic, just as this congress was not being held in the hushed, air-conditioned rooms of some Grand Hotel, but in the bare halls of a Youth Hostel. People had come from all over Europe and North America to discuss and re-read the work of an underrated, alcoholic writer who had ended up in a state of despair and general neglect, a man who had started to speak English when he was fourteen years old, son of poor Canuck immigrants, who had never learnt to speak a single sentence correctly in the language of his forbears, French, who had gone in search of his origins in Brittany, getting hopelessly mixed up with original words and place names, a writer who was to die in the most inebriate loneliness, isolated from his own buddies on the road.

Yet they were there, moved and full of enthusiasm, witnesses to that indomitable need for music, visions and fantasy, that was perhaps only by accident embodied in the figure and narrations of Ti Jean, but, in a more general way, signified the truest tribute that a man can offer to his peers: thanks for having introduced him to poetry.

In the days that follow Leo thinks about things in a way he has possibly never thought before. He thinks about the fact that his life is now inextricably bound up with writing. And he thinks that this one thing is important to him and that it is this, not himself, which is guiding the inner shifts of his life. If he did not manage to function with Thomas, if his emotional life is a mess, if, deep down, he is restless and will never find peace, it is because he is different, because he must construct a set of values that starts from the very fact that he is different. Nothing he has so far come across has gone as it should and he has been looking for the right way for years now. The fact that he is different, the things that single him out from his friends back home in the town where he was born, all this does not have to do so much with the fact that he does not have a job, or his own home, or a partner, or children. It has to do with his writing, with continually saying in words what others are quite happy to remain silent about. His sexuality, his emotional self, gamble not with other people, as he has always tended to think, ending up each time against a brick wall, but, at close quarters, with a text that does not yet exist.

He has always been ashamed and blushed, as a result, when, in the most varied of situations – on a train, or at a party, or in front of some official bureaucrat – someone has asked him what he does for a living, what job he has. He has been ashamed because he has immediately sensed that if he said 'I'm a writer' they would look at him as if he were crazy, or, in the best of scenarios, someone about to die of starvation. The difference between him and other people, his distance from others, would have seemed even more extreme. Then he would beat about the bush, inventing respectable and socially acceptable professions for himself, never that of a writer, a time-waster, a person who was of no use. Once he found himself trapped in a dinner party with a few aristocrats, industrialists, financiers and bankers. Leo was meant to be the guest of honour. Even though everybody came up and exchanged words with him, he was aware that as they shook his hand they were looking at his tie and wondering, above all, how much money he could possibly earn with such an unconventional profession. He realised that the fact that he did not have hundreds of employees at his beck and call, that he did not have estates or several houses, that he did not wield any kind of power, all this meant that he was absolutely fatuous in their eyes. A bore. One afternoon, when he found himself speaking in a small theatre on the outskirts of Milan to an audience of respectable elderly women, high-school teachers, headmistresses and the like, he suddenly broke off and was unable to find the thread of his talk. The reason was because he had had the crystal clear image of finding himself in an animal protection centre; and his audience was looking at him with that well-meaning curiosity that people have for animals that are about to become extinct. He was terrified that those little old ladies with their pastel coloured shawls and scarves would get to their feet and gently commit him to a cage and hand him little biscuits to nibble at and feed on, murmuring their endearments to make him smile and feel better. Because if the truth be told he felt that he was on the verge of extinction too.

So perhaps, throughout his life, the fact of being apart is nothing else – as Thomas had understood so well – than an elaborate setting for his own unquenchable desire to disappear; the spectacular public manifestation of a guilt complex, of an anxiety that he has perhaps felt ever since the very first day when he opened his eyes on the world, an anxiety that he would never find happiness. And this sense of guilt, at having been born, at having had a place that he did not want, at his mother's unhappiness, at the coarseness of his home town, all this has been transferred into a world apart, the world of literature, permitting him to survive and even feel gladness, but always with the consciousness that the fullness of life, as other people usually see it, would never be his for the taking. It is probably this sense of fundamental loss that has pushed him to the point where he now finds himself.

In the afternoons he spends in the Saint-Alexandre Pub, a replica of American saloons, copying the others by ordering huge bottles of Dow ale while the intellectual habitués sip at small bottles of European beer, talking nineteen to the dozen, discussing this and that with such sincerity, listening to others talking, making self-referential notes on newspapers, he feels happy, in a way. It is as if he were once more in the smoke-filled rooms of his college days. He feels the same desire to understand, and interpret, and discuss. And he sees himself mirrored in the young students who flock into the pub, quietly smoking and reading a book, writing in a notebook, staring blankly past the white curtains at the rain falling thick and fast on Rue Saint-Jean. And he thinks of Eugenio, the kid he in jest calls 'the first secretary', who goes with him on journeys and to parties, just as Thomas used to do. Leo has great confidence in Eugenio's intelligence and culture. He has been part of his life for more than a year now. One night, in the huge, comforting closeness that now existed between them which was shyly allowing desire to peek through, he said: 'You're quite right to want a permanent companion. But it can never be me.' He thinks of his group of friends, how nice they are to him when they all meet up in Florence in somebody's house and talk all night long. He knows he is important to them. They too are vital for him, because they offer him a comparison and, above all, a mirror of his dream of youth. Nothing is more of a cliché than saying: life goes on. But now he really feels this, because out there in the world he knows people who do go on.

Then all of a sudden something terribly beautiful emerges for him, too, with all the marvel of a seed that blooms after four long years of endless convalescence, years of aridity and drought and floods. He had thought he had lost this for ever, and instead, one morning, towards midday, in the Saint-Alexandre Pub, desire came back into him, reflected in a pair of blue eyes beneath a pair of thick, pale eyebrows, in a thick head of hair pulled back and slicked down with a brush, in a pair of pale corduroy Levi's and a soft grey velvet jacket. Leo looks at him and spots his slender wrists covered with light down like Hermann's, tapering fingers streaked with nicotine, a friendly, open smile, eyes narrowing the way he has liked since he was a boy. A slightly absent-minded way of rolling his cigarette, a bit ham-fisted. And the large Dow beer on the table.

When the Vondel leaves the pub Leo follows him. Their eyes meet for a second in the doorway and the man wears a slightly embarrassed expression on his face, just like Leo, as he holds out his hand, and the man takes it, without a word. Leo would just like to let him know that he was not expecting to find him there, but how could he begin to tell him about all that? Then the man lifts the collar of his jacket, winds his scarf around his neck, and walks off, hugging the walls of the houses to keep out of the wet, jumping between the puddles. Then, a hundred yards down the road, he stops, hesitates for a split second, and turns. He sees Leo outside the pub, standing in the middle of the road and looking after him. He raises a hand and waves, and Leo does the same, smiling and soaked with rain. Then the man walks on and Leo stares after him until he disappears for ever, swallowed up by the mist at the end of Rue Saint-Jean.

In a few hours he goes to Montreal airport. His plane is a small Northwest turboprop. The cabin is full of passengers and he is squeezed into a small seat, his eyes filled with the fiery colours of the maple forest below. He is happy because he has felt himself become available once again. Then he thinks of Italy, his friends, Eugenio who will come and meet him in Milan, Eugenio, for whom Leo has bought some presents . . . He follows the words of the Morrissey song: 'I'm so glad to grow older, to move away from those younger years.' He is, in a way, happy. In a few hours he will board the jumbo jet, read a few pages of a magazine, listen to some music, and drop off to sleep, then wake up a few minutes later in the dazzling light of a new day. In a few hours, in a day's time, perhaps in three or five or twenty years' time, he will feel a twinge seize him in the chest or lungs or abdomen. Although so many years have passed, or just one hour, he will remember his love and once more see Thomas's eyes, just as he saw them that last time. Then, with a resolve that is as moving as it is desperate, he will know that there is nothing more that can be done. He will go to his therapies and treatment, he will change hospital beds, but he will always know, no matter what time of day, by the grace of almighty God, that for him and his metaphysical bug, his writing, and his Vondels and Madisons, for all of them the time has come to say farewell.